BMA

Final FRCR 2B Long Cases

A Survival Guide

Final FRCR 2B Long Cases

A Survival Guide

Edited by

Jessie Aw
Austin Health, Melbourne, Australia
John Curtis
University Hospital Aintree, Liverpool, UK

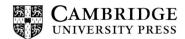

CAMBRIDGE
UNIVERSITY PRESS

University Printing House, Cambridge CB2 8BS, United Kingdom

Published in the United States of America by Cambridge University Press, New York

Cambridge University Press is part of the University of Cambridge

It furthers the University's mission by disseminating knowledge in the pursuit of
education, learning and research at the highest international levels of excellence.

www.cambridge.org
Information on this title: www.cambridge.org/9780521740692

First published 2010
5th printing 2018

Printed in the United Kingdom by Print on Demand, World Wide

A catalogue record for this publication is available from the British Library

Library of Congress Cataloging-in-Publication data

Final FRCR 2B long cases : a survival guide / edited by Jessie Aw, John Curtis.
    p. cm.
  ISBN 978-0-521-74069-2 (pbk.)
  1. Radiology, Medical–Examinations, questions, etc.   2. Radiology,
Medical–Examinations–Study guides.   3. Royal College of Radiologists
(Great Britain)–Examinations.   I. Aw, Jessie.   II. Curtis, John, 1963–   III. Title.
  RC78.15.F56 2010
  616.07′57076–dc22

                                                                    2010008975

ISBN 978-0-521-74069-2 Paperback

This book is dedicated to my parents and brothers:
Khin Khin Cho, Sein Hwat, Jack and Richard.
Jess Aw

I dedicate my work to Juliet and Matthew.
John Curtis

Contents

Contributors

Jessie Aw
Neuroradiology Fellow, Austin Health, Melbourne, Australia

Neil Collin
Specialist Registrar, Radiology, The Severn Training Scheme, Bristol, UK

John Curtis
Consultant Radiologist, University Hospital Aintree, Liverpool, UK

Indran Davagnanam
Specialist Registrar, Queens Square, London, UK

Olga Hatsiopoulou
Specialist Registrar, Radiology, Royal Liverpool University Hospital, UK

Joanna Kasznia-Brown
Specialist Registrar, Radiology, The Severn Training Scheme, Bristol, UK

Monica Khanna
Consultant Radiologist, Imperial College Healthcare NHS Trust, London, UK

Alice Pocklington
Specialist Registrar, Radiology, The Severn Training Scheme, Bristol, UK

Kate Taylor-Robinson
Paediatric Radiology Fellow, Alder Hey Children's Hospital, Liverpool, UK

Kiat Tan
Fellow in Cardiovascular MRI, University of Toronto, Toronto, Canada

Mandy Williams
Specialist Registrar, Radiology, The Severn Training Scheme, Bristol, UK

Marc Williams
Locum Consultant Radiologist, Craigavon Area Hospital, Northern Ireland

Foreword

This is a well‑presented pocket book containing a collection of imaging cases orga-
nized into the format of packets, each containing six long cases, as experienced in the
Royal College of Radiologists FRCR part 2B examination.

The collection spans a wide spectrum of pathology from common to more unusual
conditions, and provides model answers to help the candidate formulate a logical
approach and appropriate differential diagnosis for each case. A thorough review of
each final diagnosis is given, with references for further reading.

This book will be invaluable to registrars preparing for their radiology examinations, and will also serve as an excellent refresher course for consultant colleagues
who are facing the prospect of revalidation in the near future.

The authors are to be congratulated on bringing together such a diverse and
informative group of cases.

Dr Hilary Fewins MB BS FRCR
Consultant Radiologist, Liverpool Heart and Chest Hospital,
NHS Foundation Trust

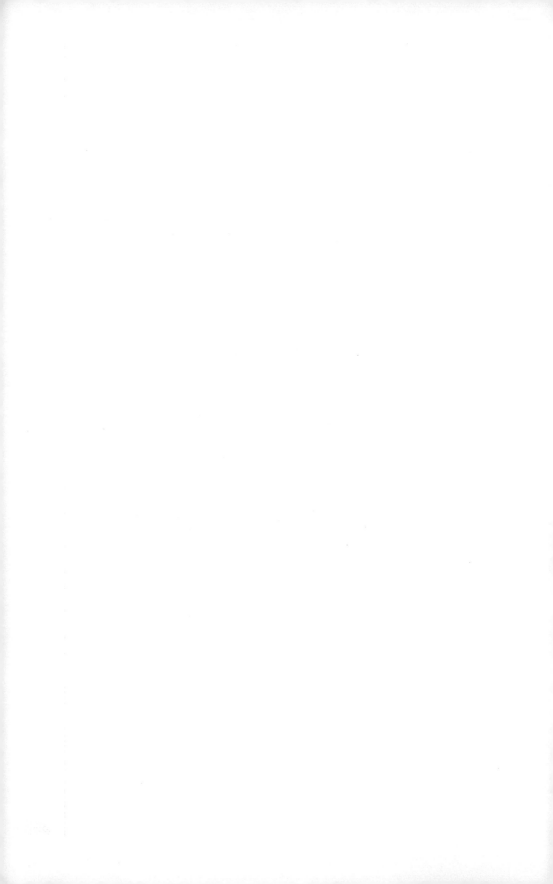

Preface

The idea for this guide came to me (JA) when I discovered a lack of suitable texts during the period I was revising for the Fellowship of the Royal College of Radiologists (FRCR) exam. I hope it will provide you with the necessary tools to enter the examination hall with full confidence and as a sound basis for your future work as a radiologist.

This book has been arranged and produced in a manner to provide a self-assessment guide to the Long Cases. In addition the book can be used as an educational book for radiology trainees during the course of their training.

In the following chapters we provide case examples, which are appropriate to the standard and level for examination. Some of the cases may be at a slightly higher level, so that you may be able to tackle situations with which you may be unfamiliar.

The chapters have been intentionally produced as heterogeneously as possible by the list of contributing authors in order to demonstrate that the cases could be answered in several ways. Each contributor has passed the exam by answering using his or her style and so we hope this book will emulate the real-life situation as well as providing an insight into the fact that there is no perfect answer for each case.

The Royal College of Radiologists has provided a suggested format, which can be the starting point and basis for tackling the exam, but as everything in life, there are no hard and fast rules. The main point is to ANSWER all the questions using a logical and safe approach in the given TIME provided.

We would like to thank all of the contributing authors for their input and hard effort. We would like to thank them for appreciating the fact that the cases have been mixed in a 'chapter' and for sharing their experiences together to bring this book to life. Jess Aw would like to thank Mr Roy Cox, Superintendent Radiographer, Basildon and Thurrock University Hospitals NHS Foundation Trust.

Jess Aw
John Curtis

Introduction

JESSIE AW

FRCR Examination Part 2B

The final examination of the Fellowship of the Royal College of Radiologists (part 2B) comprises several components:

- A rapid reporting session
- *A reporting session* (or known amongst trainees as the 'Long Cases')
- An oral examination

This guide-book will only concentrate on the reporting session. You may find the structure useful as a basis for future reporting in your practice if you so wish.

What does the *reporting session* consist of?

Currently it consists of:

- Six cases, on 'hard copy' film. In April 2010 for those sitting the examination in the UK, the Royal College of Radiologists will conduct this part of the examination and the rapid reporting section using a digital format. The viva section of the examination is likely to be in digital format in 2012. Please keep updated by visiting the Royal College website at http://www.rcr.ac.uk
- A total of 45 minutes is provided to complete writing all your answers in the booklet provided

The cases may include plain radiographs, ultrasound, radionuclide imaging, CT and MR imaging. The cases may include a mixture of cases from all the six modules with varying degrees of complexity and difficulty. Any type of the stated radiological imaging can occur and often the case can involve more than one imaging modality, e.g. a case can comprise a plain radiograph and further investigations, for example CT and radionuclide imaging. Currently the Royal College of Radiologists has not yet stated that PET or PET-CT will be included. However, this is most likely to be included in the foreseeable future. Any changes will be published on-line and can be found at http://www.rcr.ac.uk

If using 'hard copy' films, you will be provided with:

- A small table and chair
- A double viewing box
- A bright light

- A magnifying glass
- A rule
- An answer booklet to write all your cases

If using the digital format, you will be provided with:

- A small table and chair
- A computer monitor
- An answer booklet to write all your cases

Marking scheme

The marking scheme is relatively straightforward and transparent (see Table 1). However the specific criteria used to obtain the marks cannot be provided.

Each case is eligible for a maximum mark of 8 in a closed marking system. The total marks are then added up to provide a final total mark. In order to pass the reporting session comfortably, you must obtain an average of 6 out of 8 per case. You can afford to fail badly on *a single case* if you average 7 out of 8 per case. This is not advisable though.

If a candidate is on the pass/fail border for the oral component of the FRCR Clinical examinations, the marks from both the rapid reporting and reporting sessions are taken into account.

Table 1 *The marking scheme for the reporting session*

Mark	Scheme
4	Bad fail
5	Fail
6	Pass
7	Good pass
8	Excellent

Guidance and top tips to tackling the long cases

The purpose of this book is to provide some guidance and a strategy to tackle the exam. This book is not intended to be a comprehensive textbook by any means, but to be used for practising and ironing out any issues. We emphasize how important it is to be vigilant with TIMING and to be very strict about it. This is an area which the majority of individuals may not have prepared for or thought about.

All the components of the exams have to be passed and you will want to go to your viva (if you haven't done so already) in a less stressed mental frame of mind rather than worrying about what you may or may not have written for the 'long cases'.

Whatever you think about your performance in each section of the examination, it is vitally important that you stay focussed on the part of the examination that you are currently undertaking. There is no point in reminiscing about what you could have done better in the viva when you have 45 minutes to concentrate on the 'long cases'.

The following guidance notes may seem simple and obvious. However, there is good reason to reinforce these principles not only in this book but also in the guidance notes that are available from the Royal College of Radiologists' website (http://www.rcr.ac.uk). In spite of this, the guidance is not necessarily being adhered to by candidates.

The approach I have taken in this section of the exam was to place myself in the shoes of the examiner. Put yourself in this scenario: you have spent 3–5 days away from home, invigilating, examining and performing various other duties. You will be exhausted to say the least. Thereafter, you will be given a large stack of long cases to mark!

Also the report represents your ability to analyze and effectively communicate a clinically relevant opinion to all members of the clinical team. If you think in those terms then there should be minimal difficulty.

So what would the examiner marking these booklets want?

The examiner will want to finish his or her work quickly and with minimal effort.

How can you achieve this for the examiner?

- Legibility

It is very difficult to give a candidate marks if you cannot read their handwriting. How many frustrated minutes have you wasted trying to decipher a clinician's handwriting and given up?

- Neat

The booklet, if presented well, will be a pleasure for the examiner to mark.

- Structured and logical
- Concise and succinct

I have placed these two points together, as it is hard to separate them. The examiner, on behalf of the Royal College of Radiologists, will want to establish that you have a structured and logical approach to your method of dealing with each case. This will also help you structure your thoughts in the exam, when the adrenalin rush is playing havoc with your normal self.

The second point is to be concise and succinct. For this purpose, I would like to counsel you to place yourself as a clinician reading this report. Clinicians are busy and most likely will not want to read an essay, no matter how accurate and eloquent it is. On the flip side, do not be imprecise or too short. A moderate balance must be reached.

- Safe approach

Demonstrate a safe approach to the case. This must be borne in mind when you are formulating the *management* aspect to the case. Remember, the cases displayed are taken from real-life events. You must not forget about patient care and our duty as CLINICAL RADIOLOGISTS.

- Not necessary to get the absolute single correct answer in all cases

Do not waste time or get too focussed on getting the absolute right answer for an individual case at the expense of the remainder of cases. Timing for the reporting session is very important. Some of the cases may be more complex cases, which may require differential diagnosis rather than a single answer. Remember back when you may have performed a maths test, it was more important to demonstrate your abilities by displaying the analysis and deduction in solving the equation. Similarly it is crucial to display your observational skills, interpretation and deduction.

- TIMING

I cannot stress how important this aspect is. This must be practised rigorously. Each case is set out as a single exam. Inaccurate timing resulting in missing out a single case is disastrous as you will lose out on 8 marks. Once lost, this is extremely difficult to recover from. Whatever method you use, you must do all six cases in the 45 minutes. This equates to 7½ minutes per case. However, if you practise doing a case in 6 minutes, that will provide you with 9 minutes to go over the cases again or go back to any cases which you were unsure about. Clearly more complex cases will take longer and straightforward cases less time.

I would advise that if you are stuck on a case, then do not waste time on it, carry on and return to it. You will still be able to obtain marks by writing as much as possible; i.e. the examination, observations and interpretation. **NEVER LEAVE A CASE BLANK**.

- Finally, remember that the report you write would mirror what you would be expected to do in a clinically relevant report in your department every working day.

An ideal report

There is no such thing as an ideal report. However, a useful approach when tackling an examination is the following questions that you may want to ask yourself.

There are four essential elements to be answered. If you remember these questions then it provides a grounded approach, especially when the imaging may be unfamiliar to you.

1. What can be seen?
   This assesses your observational skills. This can include both normal features that are relevant to the case and abnormalities.
2. Why does it look like that?
   Once you have recognized an abnormality, you must be able to describe it so that when someone reads just the report they will be able to imagine it. This technique is also useful in the viva – describe features on the film as if the examiner were at the end of a phone and unable to see the film.
3. What has caused it?
   This question is asking about the diagnosis or possible diagnoses. It is assessing your analytical skills and whether you are able to understand what you have seen is significant or not.
4. What needs to be done next?
   Finally, this question is about what you do with your findings or management.

The clinical radiologist is pivotal in steering the clinician in providing appropriate management. This is clearly vital when an urgency arises and there is a need for urgent clinical input. This is the safe approach. Often it is the radiologist who clinches the diagnosis and provides the information necessary to allow further management to proceed.

Example of a well-presented case

Further examples of a specimen report can be found on the RCR website (http://www.rcr.ac.uk).

Question
History: haemoptysis, CTPA showed mass lesion. For staging please.

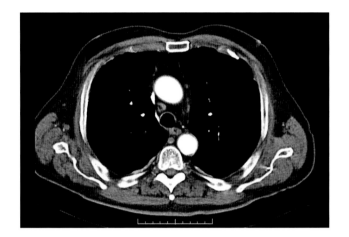

Figure I.1

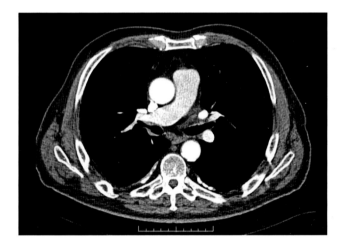

Figure I.2

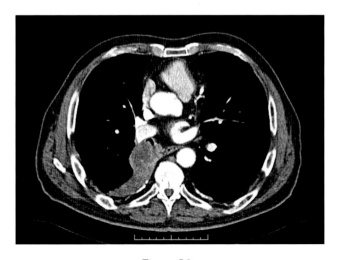

Figure I.3

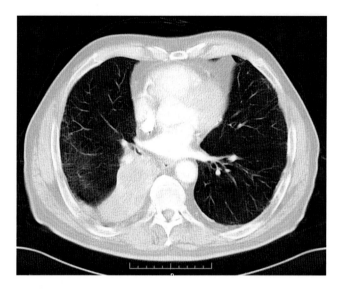

Figure I.4

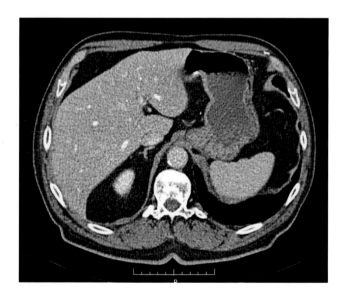

Figure I.5

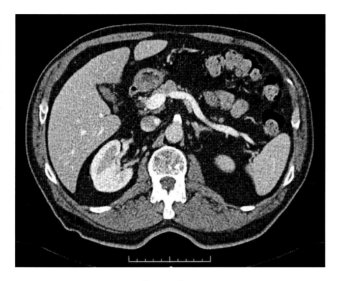

Figure I.6

Examination
- Axial CT chest and liver examination with IV contrast.

Answer

Observations and interpretations
CT chest and upper abdomen with IV contrast.

- There is luminal narrowing of the bronchus intermedius due to external compression by a soft tissue density mass.
- There is near complete obstruction of the right lower lobe bronchus also with complete collapse of the right lower lobe.
- It is difficult to delineate the soft tissue mass from the post-obstructive consolidation and associated collapse of the right lower lobe. However it is approximately greater than 3 cm in the transverse diameter.
- There is a right-sided precarinal ovoid lymph node with a fatty hilum. This is most likely a benign node.
- There is a 1 cm subcarinal lymph node, which may be significant by size criteria in this clinical context.
- Calcified pleural plaques suggestive of previous asbestos exposure.
- No supraclavicular, axillary or left hilar lymphadenopathy.
- The liver appears normal with no focal lesion.
- Both adrenal glands appear normal.
- Background generalized bilateral moderate emphysematous change with bullous formation in both lower lobes.
- Degenerative change in the axial skeleton.

Diagnosis
- Right-sided primary bronchogenic carcinoma causing complete collapse of the right lower lobe and near complete occlusion of the middle lobe bronchus with a highly suspicious subcarinal lymph node.

- This is on a background of previous asbestos exposure and generalized emphysematous change.
- There are no distant metastases.

Management
- The report needs to be **highlighted to the referring clinical team urgently** either via phone or faxing the report.
- The patient is to be discussed in the next multidisciplinary lung cancer meeting for further histological diagnosis.
- Soft tissue may be obtained via a bronchoscopy or CT guided lung biopsy depending upon the lung function and any bleeding diastheses, which will need to be reversed, e.g. warfarin therapy.

Example of an unsuitable case

Using the same case as above, the following report is issued by the candidate.

[Handwritten report:]

CT Chest with contrast

The CT chest shows a soft tissue mass in the right hilum with post obstructive consolidation of the right lower lobe

There is a mediastinal lymph node which contains a normal fatty hilum so is unlikely to be involved.

There is asbestos lung disease with COPD changes.

Normal appearance of the liver, adrenal & kidneys

Conclusion

The soft tissue mass in the Rt lung is a lung cancer

Packet 1 Case 1 Question

ALICE POCKLINGTON

Clinical history

A 51-year-old woman called for first screening in the NHS Breast Screening Programme.

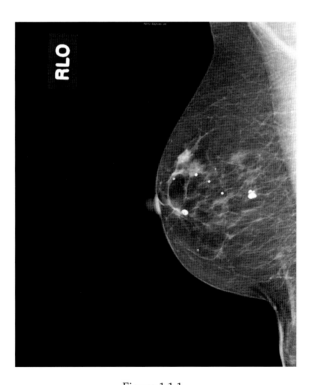

Figure 1.1.1

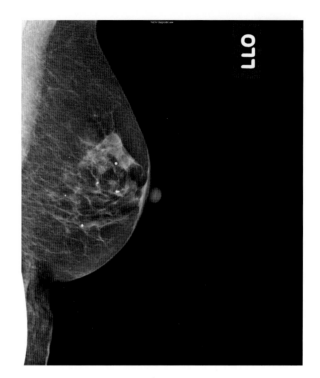

Figure 1.1.2

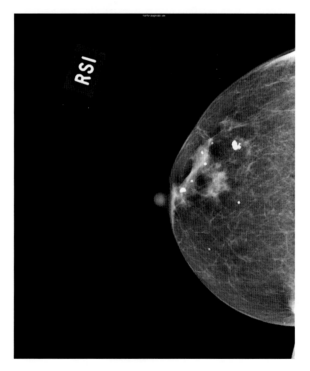

Figure 1.1.3

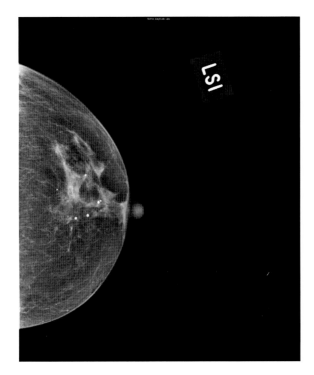

Figure 1.1.4

Packet 1 Case 1 Answer

Model answer

Examination
Standard bilateral two view mammograms; bilateral medio-lateral oblique (MLO) (Figures 1.1.1 and 1.1.2) and cranio-caudal (CC) (Figures 1.1.3 and 1.1.4) mammograms.

Findings and interpretations
- Both breasts are of principally fatty density with residual glandular tissue centrally in a symmetrical distribution.
- There are multiple well-defined flecks of calcification bilaterally. All areas are of benign appearance.

Diagnosis
Bilateral benign type breast calcification; M2.

Differential diagnosis
There are no suspicious features.

Management
No further action is required. Return to routine screening programme.

In the case above
The appearances are benign and the patient returned to routine screening.

Benign breast calcification

The National Health Service Breast Screening Programme (NHSBSP) currently calls all women aged between 50 and 70 years for bilateral mammogram every 3 years. It has been demonstrated that there is no statistical benefit in terms of mortality rates in screening more frequently than this despite an overall increase in detected total cancer rate and reduced size of tumour at the time of detection. The screening age range will gradually extend to all women aged 47 to 73 years, in order that all women

(a)   (b)

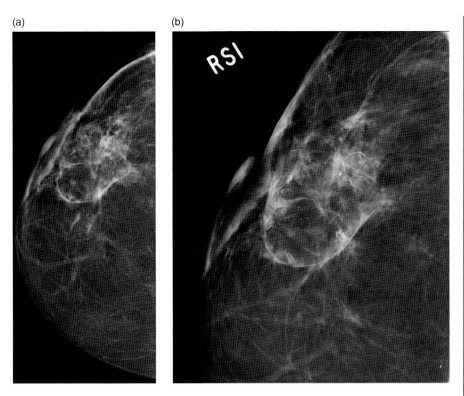

Figure 1.1.5 (a) Right cranio-caudal mammogram in a patient who has had a wide local excision for carcinoma the previous year. A few flecks of calcification are seen in the scar tissue. (b) The same view in the same patient 1 year later. There has been an increase in the number of the rounded, larger flecks of calcification. No suspicious micro-calcification.

are screened for the first time before their 50th birthday. In 2005/2006, 2.3 million women were invited to attend, with an overall acceptance rate of 75%.

All mammograms are double reported and scored M1 to M5:

- M1 is normal
- M2 benign changes only
- M3 abnormal, but probably benign
- M4 abnormal, probably malignant
- M5 malignant

Women are recalled for further assessment if reported as M3 or above. In 2005/2006, 4.7% of women were recalled. The gold standard is a recall rate of <10% for first attendees and <7% in subsequent screening rounds. This takes into account that more areas will be deemed suspicious when there are no other mammograms for comparison. Breast screening detection rate for invasive cancer is approximately 6 per 1000 women, and 1.6/1000 for in situ carcinoma.

One of the commonest findings on mammograms is breast calcification, and this must be determined to be benign, indeterminate or malignant. Anything other than benign calcification is recalled for further assessment.

The morphology and distribution of the calcification are the most important factors used to determine its nature. The commonest cause of benign calcification is fibrocystic change. Sedimented milk of calcium forms a layer in the bottom of the cyst, giving a crescentic appearance (otherwise described as 'tea-cupping') on the medio-oblique

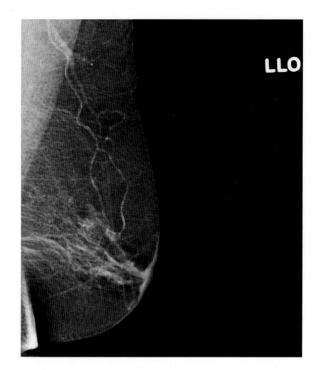

Figure 1.1.6 A left medio-lateral oblique view demonstrates benign vascular calcification in a 63-year-old woman.

view. Less commonly there is an egg-shell appearance where the cyst walls may calcify.

Smooth, rounded calcification can be due to plasma cell mastitis, fat necrosis or formed in the dilated acini of lobules. This type of benign calcification is usually more than 1 mm in diameter. It is also seen as areas of post-surgical change, which evolve over time (see Figures 1.1.5a and 1.1.5b).

Calcification within a fibroadenoma is uncommon in young women, but after the menopause it is seen as coarse popcorn-like calcification. Parallel lines of calcification are vascular in origin (Figure 1.1.6).

At each round of screening, all areas of calcification must be re-evaluated, as small foci of indeterminate or malignant calcification can easily be dismissed in a woman with previously benign calcification. Any changes should be assessed.

References

Breast Screening Frequency Trial Group. The frequency of breast cancer screening: results from the UKCCCR Randomised Trial. *Eur J Cancer* 2002; **38**: 1458–64.

Evans A, Ellis I. Breast benign calcification. In: Evans A, Pinder S, Wilson R, Ellis I, eds. *Breast calcification: a diagnostic manual*. London: Greenwich Medical Media; 2002: 4–7.

National Health Service. National Health Service Breast Screening Programme Annual Review 2007. *NHS Cancer Screening Programme* **2007**; 17.

Packet 1 Case 2 Question

INDRAN DAVAGNANAM

Clinical history

A 7-year-old male patient presenting with pyrexia, earache and a single seizure.

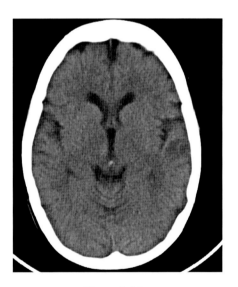

Figure 1.2.1

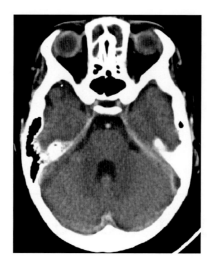

Figure 1.2.2

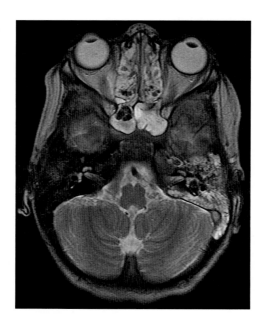

Figure 1.2.3

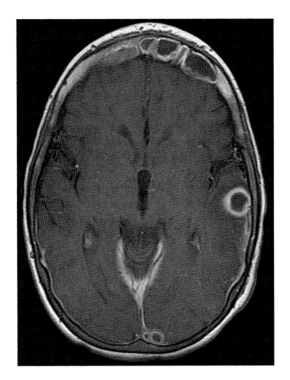

Figure 1.2.4

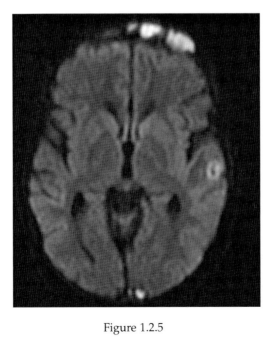

Figure 1.2.5

Packet 1 Case 2 Answer

Model answer

Examination
Pre- and post-contrast CT and MRI examinations of the cranium.

Findings
- Figure 1.2.1: Axial non-contrast CT of the brain demonstrating hypodensity in the left temporal lobe.
- Figure 1.2.2: Post-contrast axial CT of the brain showing poor opacification of the left transverse sinus and enhancement of the dura immediately adjacent to the sinus (equivalent to the 'empty-delta'sign).
- Figure 1.2.3: Axial T2-weighted image of the brain demonstrating hyperintensity of the left transverse sinus with loss of the normal flow void. There is subtotal hyperintensity of the sphenoidal, ethmoidal and left petro-mastoid air cells.
- Figure 1.2.4: Post-contrast axial T1-weighted image of the brain showing post-contrast peripheral enhancement of the left temporal lobe lesion seen on the non-contrast CT with surrounding white matter hypointensity. Lack of contrast signal is noted in the region of the posterior aspect of the superior sagittal sinus (SSS) with marked peripheral dural enhancement. There is adjacent meningeal enhancement. Left frontal sinus hypointense mucosal congestion and peripheral enhancement is also seen.
- Figure 1.2.5: Axial B1000 diffusion weighted image (DWI) demonstrating hyperintensity of the peripherally enhancing left temporal lobe lesion, SSS and left frontal sinus.

Interpretation
- Bilateral ethmoid, sphenoid and frontal sinus disease with inflammatory change.
- Left petro-mastoiditis, likely to be due to an infective aetiology.
- Left temporal lobe abscess with adjacent dural inflammation.
- Left transverse sinus and posterior SSS thrombosis.

Diagnosis
Left temporal lobe abscess and venous sinus thrombosis secondary to left mastoiditis.

Management
- Urgent referral to the paediatric neurology and neurosurgical teams.
- Contrast-enhanced MR brain review for extent of sinus thrombosis and any other focal abscesses.
- MR or CT venography.
- Intravenous antibiotic therapy and/or neurosurgical drainage.
- In non-haemorrhagic cases, anticoagulation and possibly endovascular thrombolysis of the sinus thrombus should be considered.

Cerebral abscesses and venous sinus thrombosis
Focal pyogenic abscesses of the brain are localized peripherally irregularly enhancing lesions, which typically restrict on diffusion weighted imaging, with mass effect, sulcal effacement and peripheral vasogenic oedema. These develop either from haematogeneous spread from an extracranial infective source or direct local extension from direct penetrating trauma and iatrogenic causes as well as paranasal sinus (in particular from the frontal sinus), mastoid or dental infections, spreading through the calvarium and meninges.

Patients most commonly present with headache, fever, seizures, altered mental status and focal neurological deficits. Complications such as ventriculitis, meningitis, hydrocephalus and venous sinus thrombosis arise from untreated disease or if there has been inadequate treatment.

Venous sinus thrombosis is seen on unenhanced CT as the 'delta' sign and on contrast-enhanced CT as the 'empty delta sign'. Fifty percent are associated with non-arterial territory infarction (1% of all acute strokes). Venous infarction can lead to haemorrhage in atypical locations. Both infarction and abscess restrict on diffusion weighted imaging but often the pattern of restriction of early venous infarct is heterogeneous unlike an arterial infarct and can be similar to that of an abscess.

References
Atlas S W. *Magnetic resonance imaging of the brain and spine*, Vol I, 4th edn. Lippincott, Williams & Wilkins; 2008: 863–5, 965–98.

Barkovich A J. *Pediatric neuroimaging*, 4th ed. Philadelphia: Lippincott Williams & Wilkins; 2005: 816–820 and 829–833.

Ganeshan D, Narlawar R, McCann C et al. Cerebral venous thrombosis – a pictorial review. *Eur J Radiol* 2009; doi:10.1016/j.ejrad.2009.02.07.

Osborn A G, Blaser S, Salzman K et al. *Diagnostic imaging: brain*, 1st ed. Amirsys/Elsevier; 2004: 24–27 and 96–99.

Packet 1 Case 3 Question

JOANNA KASZNIA-BROWN

Clinical history

A 2-week-old baby boy presented with a fever, dehydration and vomiting. On clinical examination he had a palpable mass in the lower part of his abdomen.

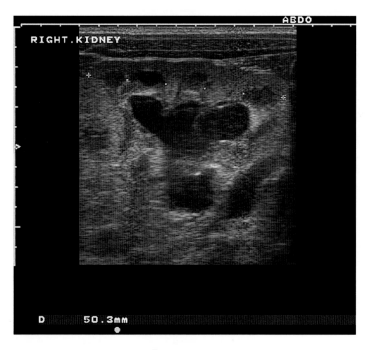

Figure 1.3.1

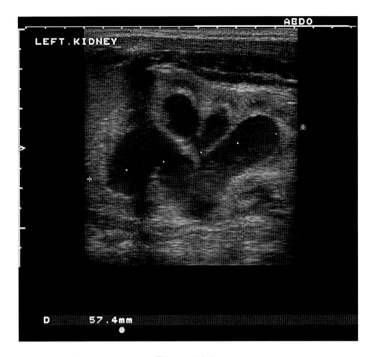

Figure 1.3.2

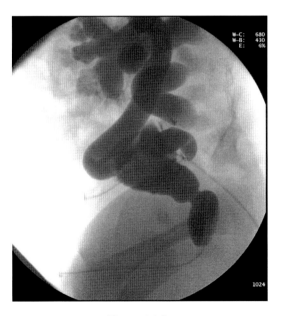

Figure 1.3.3

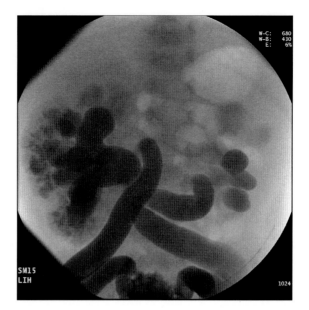

Figure 1.3.4

answer

ation
ound of the renal **tract** (Figures 1.3.1 and 1.3.2).
ating cystourethrog**ram** (MCUG) (Figures 1.3.3 and 1.3.4).

s

nd
al-sized kidneys – **the** right kidney measures 5.0 cm and left 5.7 cm.
al hydronephrosis **with** dilatation of the superior part of both ureters.

bladder with a thi**ck** and trabeculated wall.
rtrophy of bladder **neck.**
ated and dilated pos**terior** part of the urethra.
ontrast visible in the **anterior** urethra.
ral vesicoureteric refl**ux** with dilated and tortuous ureters.
ral dilatation and blu**nting** of the renal calcyces.

retation
osis +/− obstruction in the proximal urethra.
eral vesicoureteric **reflux** – grade V.
eral hydronephrosis **and** hydroureters.

osis
or urethral valves.

ential diagnosis
rior urethral valves.
aral stricture seconda**ry** to infection or trauma.
arovesical obstruction.
ary megaureter.
ive vesicoureteral refl**ux.**

Answers to follow on page 24

Pac

Mode

Exami
- Ultras
- Mictu

Findin

Ultraso
- Norn
- Bilate

MCUG
- Sma
- Hyp
- Elon
- No c
- Bilat
- Bila

Inter
1. Ste
2. Bila
3. Bila

Diag
Poster

Diffe
- An
- Ure
- Ure
- Pri
- Ma

Management

Urgent referral to the paediatric surgical/urological team.

Posterior urethral valves

Posterior urethral valves (PUVs) are a congenital abnormality related to abnormal thickening and/or fusion of the normal concentric mucosal folds (plicae colliculi) in the urethra. Valve tissue is typically very thin, but functions like a sail, causing near complete obstruction to antegrade flow of urine. It occurs exclusively in boys and is the commonest cause of urethral obstruction in children, with an incidence of 1 in 5000–8000 male births.

Three types of the valves have been described:

- Type I – most common, mucosal folds extend anteroinferiorly from the verumontanum, often fused at the lower level.
- Type II – rarest, longitudinal folds extend anterosuperiorly from the verumontanum towards the bladder neck.
- Type III – rare, diaphragm type membrane, located below verumontanum.

The clinical symptoms and presentation age are highly variable and related to the degree of the obstruction. Eight percent of diagnoses are made prenatally, 34% in the neonatal period and 32% during the first year of life.

The most common symptoms and signs include: urinary tract infection with fever and vomiting, obstructive symptoms, palpable kidneys and bladder, failure to thrive and haematuria.

Increasingly, posterior urethral valves are identified on antenatal ultrasonography; oligohydramnios, hydroureteronephrosis with dilated, thick-walled bladder (greater than 2 mm) and dilated posterior urethra are the main signs of the urethral obstruction.

Severely affected newborns may present with respiratory distress secondary to pulmonary hypoplasia, Potter facies, ascites and palpable abdominal mass. Older children can present with voiding dysfunction, urinary tract infections, sepsis, renal failure or urinary incontinence.

Ultrasound of the renal tract is the first line imaging examination. It is easily accessible and can confirm the clinical suspicion or findings from the prenatal examination. Further evaluation with MCUG is accepted as the study of choice for posterior urethral valves.

The bladder is typically distended with a thick, trabeculated wall and hypertrophy of the neck. The posterior urethra is elongated and dilated. Mucosal folds may be seen as linear lucencies, but are very often not visible. Bladder diverticula and vesicoureteric reflux are commonly present. Typically, retrograde urethrography is normal, because the retrograde flow compresses the valves against urethral wall causing a ball-valve effect.

The differential diagnosis includes: anterior urethral valves, voiding dysfunction, primary megaureter, massive vesicoureteral reflux and caecoureterocele (a ureterocele prolapsing into the posterior urethra and causing obstruction).

Complications of PUV include:

- neonatal urine leak with ascites
- pulmonary hypoplasia with pneumothorax/pneumomediastinum
- renal dysplasia.

Prognosis depends on duration of the obstruction prior to corrective surgery and the degree of renal dysplasia. Poor prognosis is associated with vesicoureteral reflux.

Treatment of PUV in children is based on endoscopic ablation of the valves. Obstetric management includes induction of labour if PUVs are diagnosed during the last 10 weeks of pregnancy and the baby is mature enough to survive. Fetal surgery is performed in cases of severe oligohydramnios with a percutaneous placement of a vesico-amniotic shunt.

References

Glassberg K I, Horowitz M. Urethral valve and other anomalies of the male urethra. In: Belman A B, King L R, Kramer S A, eds. *Clinical paediatric urology*, 4th ed. London: Martin Dunitz Ltd; 2002: 899–946.

Krishnan A, de Souza A, Konijeti R, Baskin L S. The anatomy and embryology of posterior urethral valves. *J Urol* 2006; **175**(4): 1214–20.

Packet 1 Case 4 Question

MARC WILLIAMS

Clinical history

A 23-year-old male presents with acute onset of shortness of breath and haemoptysis.

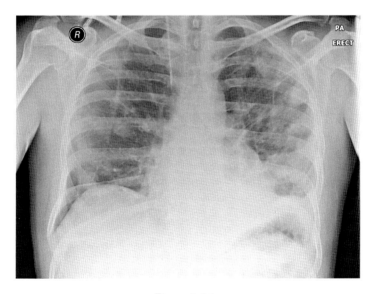

Figure 1.4.1

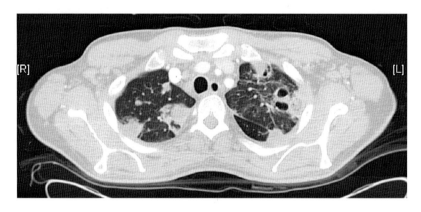

Figure 1.4.2

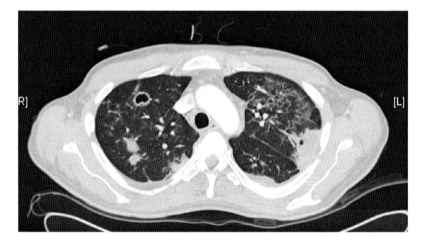

Figure 1.4.3

Answers to follow on page 30

Packet 1 Case 4 Answer

Model answer

Examination
- A chest radiograph of an adult male.
- Axial images of a CT chest.

Observations and interpretations
- The PA chest radiograph (Figure 1.4.1) demonstrates multiple small nodular opacities in both lungs, predominantly in the periphery of the left lung. Lesions in both mid zones demonstrate cavitation. The lung volumes are maintained.
- There is associated pleural opacification at the left lung base, which may represent pleural fluid or thickening.
- There is a right-sided internal jugular line, which appears well placed. No pneumothorax is visible.

Figures 1.4.2 and 1.4.3 are selected axial images from the upper zones of a CT chest examination (lung windows) demonstrating multiple nodular opacities, predominantly in the periphery of both lungs. Some of these opacities are thick-walled cavitating lesions with associated architectural distortion. There are multiple other opacities which are wedge shaped and pleurally based and may represent pulmonary infarcts.

Principal diagnosis and differential diagnosis
There is a differential diagnosis for the appearance of multiple, cavitating lung nodules though the more likely possibilities can be identified when taking into account the patient's age (malignant disease is less likely in a patient of this age).
Diagnoses to consider include:

- Multiple pulmonary infarcts (particularly in view of the pleurally based opacities). In the presence of pulmonary artery dilatation, this makes infarcts much more likely
- Septic pulmonary emboli (in a patient with symptoms and signs of bacterial infection) due to, for example, *Staphylococcus aureus* or *Klebsiella*
- Wegener's granulomatosis
- Metastatic squamous cell carcinoma
- Rheumatoid nodules

The latter two diagnoses would be less likely in view of the patient's age.

Management

The patient should be admitted to hospital (if not already there) and urgently referred to a respiratory physician.

In this case, the diagnosis is Wegener's granulomatosis. This had previously been diagnosed on the basis of blood tests (anti-neutrophil cytoplasmic antibody, ANCA), radiological features and microscopic haematuria.

Wegener's granulomatosis

A brief review of Wegener's granulomatosis will be presented with particular reference to the thoracic features of the condition.

Wegener's granulomatosis is a multisystem disease of unknown aetiology which is characterized by necrotizing granulomatous inflammation of small vessel walls resulting in necrosis and haemorrhage. It primarily affects the lungs but other areas are involved; renal tract, skin, joints, orbits and the central nervous system can be affected. In the lungs, it leads to granulomata formation and cavitating lesions. Glomerulonephritis and small vessel vasculitis can also occur. Lung involvement occurs in more than 90% of cases and renal involvement in approximately 83% of cases, which if untreated, can cause death from renal failure within months. It most commonly affects patients in the 30–60 years age group.

Respiratory symptoms are present in most individuals and include cough, dyspnoea, haemoptysis, hoarseness and stridor. Symptoms can also be caused by sinus disease or the presentation may be non-specific with symptoms of fever, malaise, arthralgia, anorexia, haematuria, proteinuria and weight loss. Vasculitis can manifest as peripheral or central mononeuropathies.

Most patients are initially investigated with a chest radiograph. A CT scan of the chest may then be undertaken to further delineate the abnormalities or to demonstrate occult findings (occasionally chest radiographs are normal). The imaging findings include:

- Most commonly, focal opacities that vary in size to include nodules and consolidation (see below) which may coexist. Nodules may vary in size and can measure up to 10 cm, though are usually 2–4 cm in size. They are usually multiple but may be single, can be thin- or thick-walled and up to 50% may cavitate. The cavity wall tends to become thinner with time. Secondarily infected nodules may have an air-fluid level. On high resolution CT, nodules may have a halo of ground glass shadowing, due to haemorrhage.
- Airspace opacification can be bilateral and diffuse or localized, with ill-defined margins due to pulmonary haemorrhage.
- Subpleural and wedge-shaped consolidation may be due to granulomata or pneumonia.
- Pleural thickening and small effusions may occur.

Confirmation of the diagnosis may be achieved by combinations of history, biopsy or laboratory evaluation (c-ANCA). It is worthy of note that c-ANCA is less often present when Wegener's granulomatosis is confined to the lungs.

References

Allen S D, Harvey C J. Imaging of Wegener's granulomatosis. *Br J Radiol* 2007; **80**: 757–65.
Dahnert W. *Radiology review manual*. Philadelphia: Lippincott, Williams & Wilkins; 2003: 534.
Ravenel J G, Irshad A. *Wegener granulomatosis, thoracic*. Updated 21 Oct, 2008; available at: http://www.emedicine.com/radio/topic743.htm

Packet 1 Case 5 Question

MANDY WILLIAMS

Clinical history

A 75-year-old female smoker presents with a 6-hour history of severe abdominal pain. On examination the abdomen was soft. Biochemistry showed an elevated lactate and acidosis.

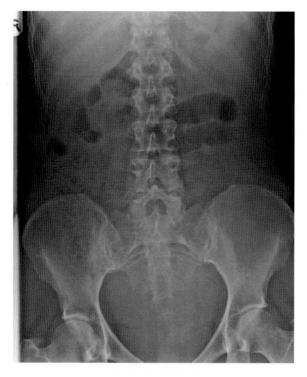

Figure 1.5.1

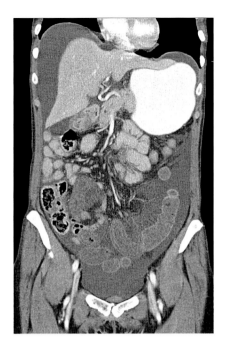

Figure 1.5.2

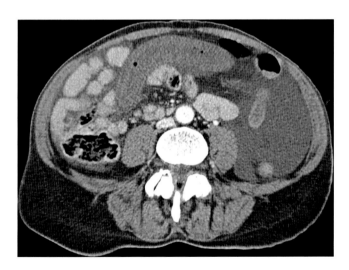

Figure 1.5.3

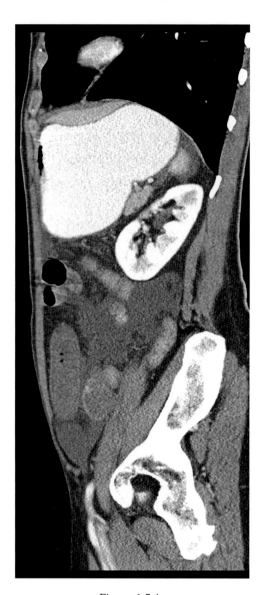

Figure 1.5.4

Answers to follow on page 36

Packet 1 Case 5 Answer

Model answer

Examination
- Plain radiograph of the abdomen.
- CT scan abdomen and pelvis post oral and IV contrast – coronal, axial and sagittal images.

Observations and interpretations
- **Plain film:** there is a dilated loop of small bowel in the mid abdomen. There is no gas seen in the large bowel. The caecum contains faeces. No free intraperitoneal gas.
- There is a large soft tissue density in the pelvis – possibly free fluid or a distended bladder. The latter is less likely as the superior border is not visualized.
- **CT:** There is a large volume of free fluid/ascites seen surrounding the liver and spleen and within the pelvis.
- There is a very oedematous loop of small bowel in the left iliac fossa and pelvis. The bowel wall in this segment is not enhancing well compared to the remainder of the small bowel.
- On the coronal images the marginal arteries are not filled with contrast.

This indicates bowel ischaemia. In the early stages there is no gas within the bowel wall and no free gas (which are late features).

Diagnosis
Small bowel ischaemia.

Differential diagnosis
- Lymphoma.
- Radiotherapy.
- Crohn's disease.
- Amyloidosis.

Management
The patient needs an urgent surgical review and resection of the ischaemic bowel.

Small bowel ischaemia

Bowel obstruction is a common presentation to both the surgical and emergency departments. The signs and presenting symptoms are usually non-specific, with early diagnosis being the key to avoid bowel necrosis and mortality. Any delay in diagnosis will increase morbidity and mortality.

There are numerous more common causes of bowel obstruction: adhesions, tumour (primary or recurrence), anastomotic stricture, inflammatory bowel disease or paralytic ileus. Ischaemia is secondary to thromboembolism in 50% of cases. Other causes include bowel obstruction, volvulus, neoplasm, vasculitis, radiotherapy and trauma.

Plain film – this may be normal in the early stages.

In this patient the main clue was in the history as she had known risk factors and metabolic acidosis on presentation. Beware of patients with **severe** pain and a **soft** abdomen.

As the bowel becomes more ischaemic there will be dilatation of the ischaemic segment of bowel. Perforation is a very late finding.

CT: post IV contrast

There are many imaging features of small bowel ischaemia. The reported sensitivity of CT in the diagnosis of ischaemia is in the range of 76–100%. The sensitivity increases when two or more signs are present. Arterial phase CT has been shown to be helpful in the diagnosis. This may not be the case if a patient presents either with other non-specific symptoms or trauma, then a different protocol is carried out to maximize the presence of bowel wall enhancement.

Imaging features include:

- Bowel wall thickening. Bowel wall thickening alone is non-specific and limited in value.
- Intramural pneumatosis. Gas bubbles in the intestinal lumen must not be confused with intramural pneumatosis.
- Mesenteric venous engorgement and/or thrombus in the mesenteric arteries.
- Reduced bowel wall enhancement: continuous or segmental reduced enhancement. This has been shown to be highly accurate in identifying small bowel ischaemia.
- Small bowel faeces sign.
- Ascites.
- Portal venous gas is seen as a late finding.

References

Chapman S, Nakielny R. *Aids to radiological differential diagnosis*, 5th ed. Edinburgh: Saunders; 2003.

Rha S E, Ha H K, Lee S H et al. CT and MR imaging findings of bowel ischaemia from various primary causes. *RadioGraphics* 2000; **20**: 29–42.

Segatto E, Mortele H, Weissner W et al. Acute small bowel ischaemia: CT imaging findings. *Seminars in Ultrasound, CT and MRI* 2003; **24**(5): 364–76.

Packet 1 Case 6 Question

KIAT TAN

Clinical history

A 70-year-old female known to have a chronic severe benign oesophageal stricture due to acid reflux presents with a 1-day history of central abdominal pain and vomiting.

(a)

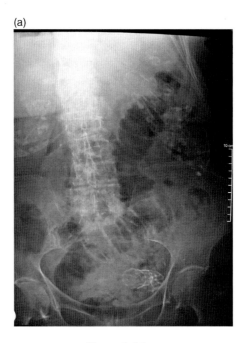

Figure 1.6.1a

Answers to follow on page 40

Packet 1 Case 6 Answer

Model answer

Examination
Plain abdominal radiograph.

Findings and interpretations
- Dilated loops of small bowel with a maximal diameter of around 5 cm (note scale to the right of image; Figure 1.6.1a).
- No large bowel dilatation.
- There is a metallic tubular density with a lattice-like appearance in the left iliac fossa. No intra-abdominal calcification.
- No free or intramural gas.
- No gas in the biliary tree.
- No stent seen in the lower oesophagus.
- Incidental degenerative changes are noted in the lower thoracic and lumbar spine.

Diagnosis

Small bowel obstruction
The finding of the metallic density on the abdominal radiograph and the history of oesophageal stricture suggest that this may be due to migration of an oesophageal stent.

Differential diagnosis
Adhesions from previous abdominal surgery and rectal stent in situ.

Management
(1) The case needs to be discussed urgently with the general surgical team as the large diameter of the small bowel indicates imminent perforation.
(2) A history of a previous oesophageal stent would clinch the diagnosis of stent ileus and comparison with prior imaging will confirm the diagnosis of stent migration if the oesophageal stent is no longer present.
(3) An urgent CT scan of the abdomen and pelvis could provide important anatomical delineation for the surgical team, confirm the diagnosis and help rule out perforation.
(4) A chest radiograph is required for pre-operative assessment and for the detection of intraperitoneal free gas (if a CT scan is not performed).

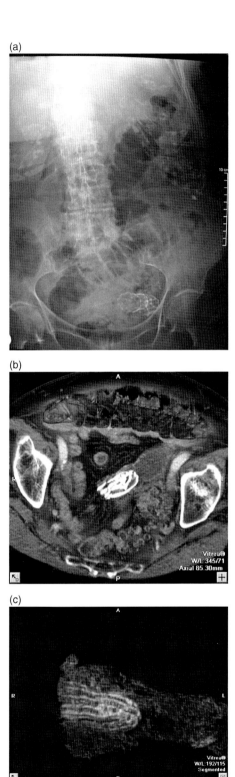

Figure 1.6.1a, b and c

Stent migration

Migration of an oesophageal stent is common, occurring in up to 35% of treated patients. Stents placed across the gastroesophageal junction and covered stents are particularly prone to migration. This is the main reason that stent placement is usually carried out on those patients with malignant disease.

A 'wait and see' approach is often reasonable in asymptomatic patients as the migrated stent often passes spontaneously per rectum. Stents in the stomach can sometimes be retrieved endoscopically.

Complications of stent migration include bowel perforation and obstruction. These complications are associated with high rates of mortality and morbidity, even with surgery. Open surgical removal of the stent is almost always required in these cases.

In the case above, the presence of stent ileus was confirmed by CT (Figures 1.6.1b and c). The stent was successfully removed at laparotomy. Unfortunately, the patient succumbed to pneumonia after the operation.

References

Hramiec J C, O'Shea M A, Quinlan R M. Expandable metallic oesophageal stents in benign disease: a cause for concern. *Surg Laparosc Endosc* 1998; **8**: 40–3.

Morgan R, Adam A. Use of metallic stents and balloons in the oesophagus and gastrointestinal tract. *J Vasc Interv Radiol* 2001; **12**: 283–97.

Packet 2 Case 1 Question

JOANNA KASZNIA-BROWN

Clinical history

A 56-year-old woman with progressive dysphagia with a past medical history of gastroesophageal reflux disease.

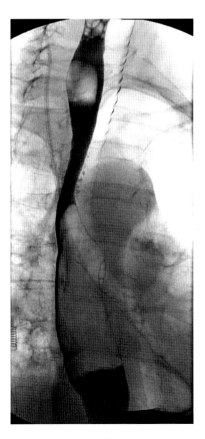

Figure 2.1.1

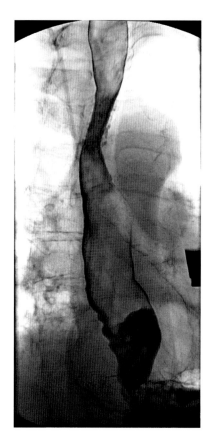

Figure 2.1.2

Answers to follow on page 46

Packet 2 Case 1 Answer

Model answer

Examination
Contrast swallow.

Findings and interpretations
- Narrowing of the lumen in the mid aspect of the oesophagus.
- Multiple flask-shaped out-pouchings of the contrast at a right angle to the oesophageal lumen. These measure 3–4 mm and communicate with the lumen through a narrow neck.
- No other mucosal irregularity.
- Moderate dilatation of the featureless lower part of the oesophagus. Tertiary peristalsis and delay in opening of the gastro-oesophageal junction.
- Thin line of contrast along the anterior wall of the trachea, consistent with aspiration of small amount of contrast into the respiratory tree.

Diagnosis
- Oesophageal intramural pseudodiverticulosis.
- Stricture in mid oesophagus (most likely of peptic origin, given the past medical history of gastro-oesophageal disease) and decreased oesophageal motility.
- Aspiration.

Management
- Urgent referral to surgical/gastroenterology team.
- Endoscopy with a biopsy to exclude/confirm *Candida* infection.
- Consider endoscopic dilatation of the oesophagus.

Oesophageal intramural pseudodiverticulosis

Oesophageal intramural pseudodiverticulosis is a rare benign disorder, occurring at all ages and more frequently in males.

The aetiology is explained by pathological dilatation of the pre-existing excretory ducts of the submucous glands. This is due to an increase in intraluminal pressure in the oesophagus and submucosal inflammation and fibrosis, secondary to chronic oesophagitis.

The condition usually presents with dysphagia; typically this is not severe and is usually intermittent and slowly progressive. There is a high incidence of oesophageal narrowing, usually in the upper third of the oesophagus associated with the 1–4 mm flask-shaped diverticula seen on the barium swallow. The diverticula usually project at right angles to the lumen and communicate via narrow-necked openings. CT shows thickening of the oesophageal wall, diffuse irregularity of the lumen and intramural gas collections.

Oesophageal pseudodiverticulosis is associated with *Candida* infection, gastro-oesophageal reflux, hiatus hernia, oesophageal dysmotility, diabetes mellitus and carcinoma.

References

Costello DAE, Choudhury R, Sherman DIN, Abramovich S. Two cases of oesophageal intramural pseudodiverticulosis. *Otorhinolaryngology, Head and Neck Surgery* 2004; 8(1): 29–31.
Sabaratnam S, Fayek DS, Morgan WE. Oesophageal intramural pseudodiverticulosis. *Thorax* 1985; **40**: 849–57.

Packet 2 Case 2 Question

ALICE POCKLINGTON

Clinical history

A 52-year-old woman presents with bilateral 'lumpy breasts'.

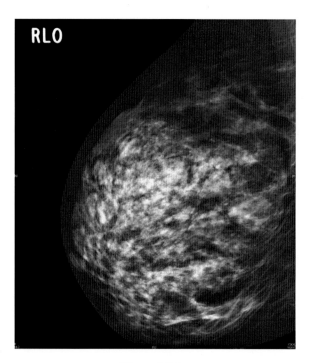

Figure 2.2.1

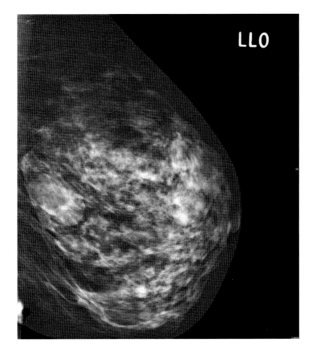

Figure 2.2.2

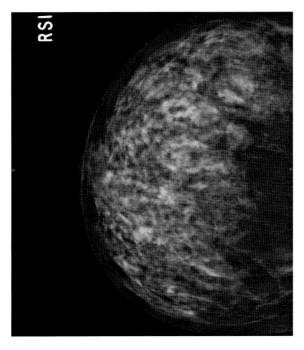

Figure 2.2.3

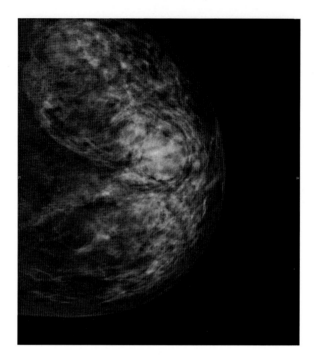

Figure 2.2.4

Answers to follow on page 52

Packet 2 Case 2 Answer

Model answer

Examination
Standard bilateral two view mammograms: bilateral medio-lateral oblique (MLO) (Figures 2.2.1 and 2.2.2) and cranio-caudal (CC) (Figures 2.2.3 and 2.2.4) mammograms.

Findings and interpretations
- Both breasts are of principally glandular density.
- Multiple well-defined rounded opacities in both breasts.
- The largest is in the central left breast and measures 2 cm in diameter (*a rule is provided in the exam*).
- No calcification.

Diagnosis
Multiple breast cysts – M2 bilateral.

Differential diagnosis
Multiple fibroadenomata.

Management
- Confirm the presence of cysts with ultrasound examination.
- If they have the appearance of simple cysts then no further action is required.
- Aspiration of large cysts can be performed with or without ultrasound guidance.
- Cyst fluid should be sent for pathological analysis if bloodstained or if the cyst does not aspirate to extinction.

In the case above
In this case the diagnosis was multiple, bilateral simple breast cysts. This was confirmed with ultrasound. No further action taken.

Breast cysts

Breast cysts are a non-proliferative benign breast lesion and are derived from the terminal duct lobule.

(a)

(b)

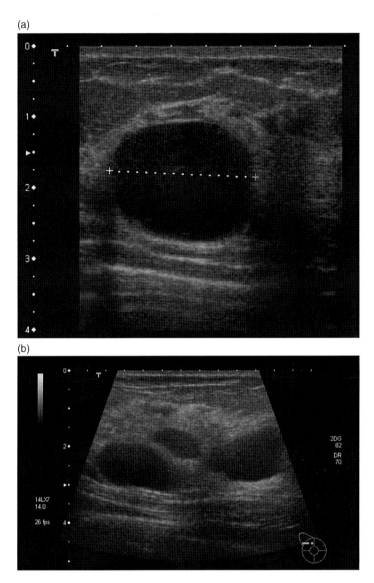

Figure 2.2.5 (a) Ultrasound image of the left breast demonstrates a well-defined, rounded, anechoic mass lesion with post-acoustic enhancement. (b) Ultrasound image of the right breast demonstrates the presence of multiple cysts in the right breast.

They are the most common cause of breast lumps in women aged 35–55 years. They are most common in the peri-menopausal period, and uncommon in post-menopausal women, in the absence of hormone replacement therapy. They are often bilateral and multiple.

Simple breast cysts are well defined and rounded if tensely filled, whilst flat cysts may not be palpable. They are variable in size, and may fluctuate in size according to the menstrual cycle. Simple breast cysts have a characteristic sonographic appearance, with 98–100% diagnostic accuracy.

A simple cyst should be round or ovoid and well circumscribed. It should also be anechoic, with post-acoustic enhancement (see Figure 2.2.5a). This allows them to be easily distinguished from other benign lesions, which have a similar mammographic

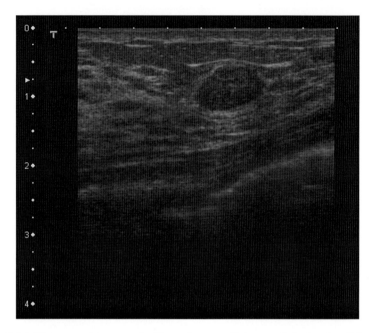

Figure 2.2.6 Ultrasound image of a fibroadenoma. It is a well-defined, solid, hypoechoic mass lesion, in comparison to an anechoic cyst.

appearance. The differential mammographic appearance for simple breast cysts is a fibroadenoma. In comparison, sonographically, a fibroadenoma is a solid hypoechoic mass lesion (see Figure 2.2.6).

Correlation should be made with the mammographic appearances regarding size, shape and position to make sure that the lesions correspond. If there is any doubt, then the cyst should be aspirated and a post-aspiration mammogram obtained.

A complex cyst is one that has any other features beyond simple cyst, i.e. thick-walled, internal echoes, bloody aspirate and does not aspirate to extinction. In this situation, a core biopsy should be performed, as 0.3% of carcinomas are intracystic.

References

Dahnert W. *Radiology review manual*, 5th ed. Lippincott, Williams & Wilkins; 2003: 556.
Harris JR, Lippman ME, Morrow M, Osborne CK. *Diseases of the breast*, 3rd ed. Philadelphia: Lippincott, Williams & Wilkins; 2004: 77.
Lindfors KK, Le-Petross HT. Breast imaging. In: Brant WE & Helms CA, eds. *Fundamentals of diagnostic radiology*, 3rd ed. Lippincott, Williams & Wilkins; 2007: 575–6.

Packet 2 Case 3 Question

MARC WILLIAMS

Clinical history

A 31-year-old female presents with right iliac fossa pain.

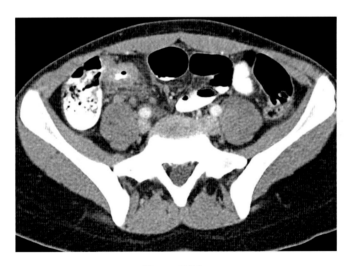

Figure 2.3.1

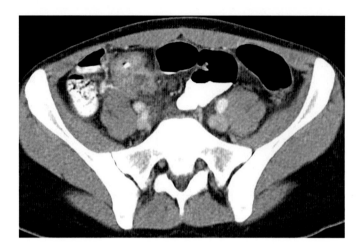

Figure 2.3.2

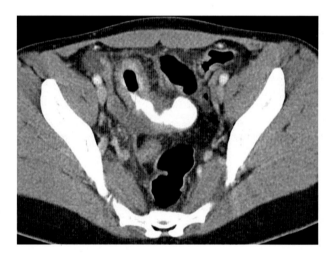

Figure 2.3.3

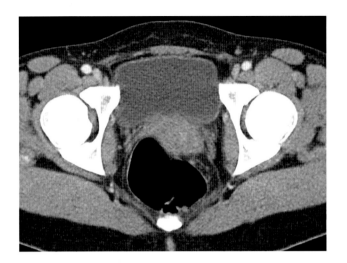

Figure 2.3.4

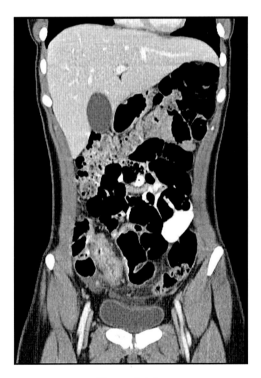

Figure 2.3.5

Packet 2 Case 3 Answer

Model answer

Examination
CT scan of the abdomen and pelvis post IV and oral contrast.

Observations and interpretations
- In the right lower quadrant, and extending into the pelvis, there is a loop of thick-walled small bowel adjacent to the caecum, which is likely to represent terminal ileum. There is associated perimesenteric stranding consistent with inflammatory changes. No local nodularity in the adjacent mesentery.
- The remainder of the visualized small and large bowel appears grossly normal. In particular there are no fluid-filled dilated bowel loops or signs of obstruction. No other focal thickening, abnormal enhancement or transitional zone is seen.
- No free intra-abdominal fluid is demonstrated.
- No free intra-abdominal gas is demonstrated.
- There are no other features of note and in particular, the visualized portions of the sacroiliac joints appear normal with no features of sacroiliitis.

Principal diagnosis and differential diagnosis
There is a differential diagnosis for the appearance of a thick-walled terminal ileum. Diagnoses which should be considered include:

- Crohn's disease: in this case, the patient may have chronic symptoms of abdominal pain, weight loss and diarrhoea.
- Lymphoma: this can have a very similar imaging appearance to Crohn's disease.
- Tuberculosis: this primarily involves the caecum giving rise to caecal contraction, i.e. the 'coned' caecum.
- *Yersinia*: no evidence of deep ulceration and resolves spontaneously.

The favoured diagnosis is inflammatory bowel disease, Crohn's disease.

Management
The report for the patient should be urgently faxed or phoned through to the referring clinician. Then the patient requires urgent referral to a gastroenterologist by the referring clinician.

Further imaging of the small bowel to identify multiple lesions can be undertaken with a small bowel meal, small bowel meal and follow through or CT/MR enteroclysis when the disease activity is indolent.

In this case
The diagnosis was Crohn's disease, which was made by biopsy.

Crohn's disease

Crohn's disease is an idiopathic, chronic, transmural inflammatory process with mucosal damage of the bowel that often leads to fibrosis and obstructive symptoms. The aetiology is unclear although genetic, infectious, altered immunology, diet, vascular abnormalities and psychological factors have all been implicated. It can affect any part of the GI tract from the mouth to the anus with presence of non-caseating granulomas and additional systemic features in some patients.

Crohn's disease has a bimodal distribution and in older patients, tends to involve the colon. It is more common in developed Western countries. Similarly with ulcerative colitis and in comparison with the general population, the cancer risk is higher in both the small and large bowel. Gastrointestinal cancer is a leading cause of mortality in long-standing Crohn's disease. The disease tends to present in one of three distinct anatomical patterns: small bowel involvement only (30%), distal small bowel and colonic involvement (45%) and colonic involvement only (25%). Small bowel involvement is found most frequently on the mesenteric border of the terminal ileum.

Clinical symptoms include fever, abdominal pain, diarrhoea and weight loss. Rectal bleeding is less common than in ulcerative colitis. Anorectal complications include fistulae, fissures and perirectal abscess. In long-standing disease, as fibrosis develops, diarrhoea decreases and obstruction may occur.

Extraintestinal manifestations include oral aphthous ulceration, erythema nodosum, avascular necrosis secondary to chronic steroid therapy, gallstone formation (due to reduced bile salt reabsorption in the terminal ileum), oxalate kidney stones, primary sclerosing cholangitis, cholangiocarcinoma, sacroiliitis (bilateral and symmetrical) and synovitis (in particular affecting lower limb joints, hands and wrists). Osteomalacia and anaemia may occur due to malabsorption. Sclerosing cholangitis and cholangiocarcinoma are more likely to be associated with ulcerative colitis than Crohn's disease.

The imaging features of Crohn's disease will be briefly discussed.

Plain radiographs can be used in the acute setting to evaluate for bowel obstruction; bowel wall oedema and an empty collapsed bowel imply active colitis. Of importance is the exclusion of toxic megacolon and pneumoperitoneum which is an acute surgical emergency. In long-standing disease there may be fusion of the sacroiliac joints, gallstones and signs to suggest the possibility of metastases from an occult colonic carcinoma. Patients with Crohn's disease have an increased incidence of a cancer of the gastrointestinal tract compared with the general population.

Double contrast studies are still the gold standard to demonstrate aphthoid ulceration in early Crohn's disease. The ulcers are seen as punctate collections of barium surrounded by a radiolucent halo due to surrounding mucosal oedema. There may be intervening normal mucosa, which leads to skin lesions. In contrast to ulcerative colitis, Crohn's disease is characterized by a fine granular appearance to the mucosa with disease extension proximally either for a short segment or continuously from the rectum, the extent of which may lead to a pancolitis.

As more severe Crohn's disease develops, the small ulcers enlarge, become more confluent and extend deeper into the bowel wall forming clefts which gives the appearance of cobblestoning, i.e. ulceration surrounding rounded normal islands of mucosa. In long-standing disease, transmural inflammation leads to stricture formation which gives rise to the string sign of Kantor that is often seen in the terminal ileum. Intestinal obstruction may occur as a consequence. Inflammation may extend through the bowel wall into the surrounding mesentery leading to sinuses, fistulae and abscess formation.

Mucosal ulceration can also be detected on multidetector CT using a high-resolution protocol with fine cuts, although small bowel contrast examinations or enteroclysis studies are more sensitive for the early mucosal changes of Crohn's disease. The advantage of CT is in the detection of transmural changes, the extra-intestinal and intraperitoneal pathology of Crohn's disease, i.e. abscesses and fistulae.

The CT findings of Crohn's disease include bowel wall thickening, mesenteric stranding, an increase in mesenteric fat ('creeping fat'), local lympadenopathy, fistu-lae, inflammatory masses and abscesses. Contrast examinations may be more sensi-tive than CT in demonstrating a fistulous track but CT is more readily able to depict the consequences of the fistula, for example air in the bladder. In the acute situation, CT is the modality of choice to determine the diagnosis even in patients with known diagnoses of inflammatory bowel disease. It will demonstrate any associated compli-cations in order to assist with management decisions. CT is also highly valuable in assisting for detection of carcinoma of the small bowel (adenocarcinoma and small bowel lymphoma) especially after bypass surgery, where it is difficult to adequately image with barium studies and unfeasible with colonoscopy.

MRI is an emerging technique with its high soft tissue contrast and the lack of ionizing radiation is a positive advantage over CT, especially in the long-term follow-up situations.

MRI has a particular role in the evaluation of the anorectal complications of Crohn's disease, i.e. sinus tracks and fistulae, which often appear hyperintense on T2-weighted images (preferably with fat suppression) because of their fluid content. The relationship of the fistulous track to the levator ani muscle is of particular surgical importance. MRI also readily demonstrates abscess formation.

References

Chen Y-H, Zhou D. *Crohn disease*. 26 Jan 2007; available at: http://www.emedicine.com/radio/TOPIC197.HTM

Dahnert W. *Radiology review manual*. Philadelphia: Lippincott, Williams & Wilkins; 2003: 809–10.

Furukawa A, Saotome T, Yamasaki M et al. Cross-sectional imaging in Crohn disease. *RadioGraphics* 2004; **24**: 689–702.

Gore RM, Balthazar EJ, Ghahremani GG, Miller FH. CT features of ulcerative colitis and Crohn's disease. *AJR* 1996; **167**: 3–15.

Packet 2 Case 4 Question

KIAT TAN

Clinical history

A 50-year-old patient presenting with acute-on-chronic abdominal pain.

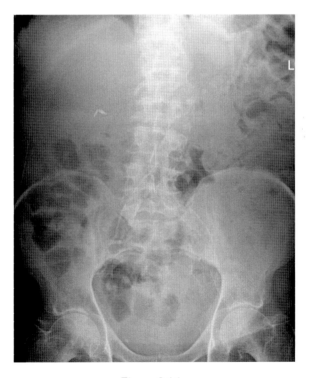

Figure 2.4.1

Packet 2 Case 4 Answer

Model answer

Examination
Plain abdominal radiograph.

Findings and interpretations
- Surgical clips in right upper quadrant.
- Speckled calcification extending from the epigastrium to the left hypochondrium.
- Dense aortic, iliac and femoral calcification.
- Bowel gas pattern is unremarkable.
- No free gas.
- No intramural gas.
- No gas in the biliary tree.
- Degenerative changes noted in the spine.

Diagnosis
Pancreatic calcification due to chronic pancreatitis most probably due to alcohol abuse and probably secondary diabetes.

Differential diagnosis
- Chronic pancreatitis due to cholelithiasis.
- Diabetic ketoacidosis can also present with acute abdominal pain.

Management
(1) Discuss with surgeons.
(2) Need to rule out diabetic ketoacidosis.
(3) Further imaging required.

An ultrasound should be obtained in the first instance to detect possible common bile duct stones and complications: pseudocysts/abscesses. A CT scan may also be required.

Chronic calcific pancreatitis

Chronic pancreatitis is the result of repeated episodes of acute pancreatitis due to a range of causes. Major predisposing risk factors for chronic pancreatitis may be categorized with the TIGAR-O system; Toxic-metabolic (smoking/alcohol/diet), Idiopathic (Tropical calcific pancreatitis), Genetic (cystic fibrosis gene, serine protease inhibitor Kazal type 1 and cationic trypsinogen gene), Autoimmune, Recurrent and severe acute pancreatitis (post-necrotic, vascular) or Obstructive (pancreatic divisum).

Chronic calcific pancreatitis due to alcohol abuse has been reported in 20–40% of cases and usually develops after 5–10 years of repeated attacks of acute pancreatitis. The 'rosary crown' appearance has been described for the changes of the main pancreatic duct induced by alcohol. It describes areas of stenosis alternating areas of dilatation with background parenchymal fibrosis, architectural distortion related to traction fibrosis. Tropical calcific pancreatitis (a type of idiopathic chronic pancreatitis occurring in tropical regions), hyperparathyroidism and hereditary pancreatitis are also associated with pancreatic calcification. Pancreatic calcification is rare in pancreatitis due to cholelithiasis. In the FRCR examination (and after!) always look for associated radiological signs that may suggest a unifying diagnosis such as hyperparathyroidism. The presence of renal stones may link with calcification of the pancreas in such cases as renal papillary necrosis due to alcohol or diabetes.

Gross vascular calcification is unusual in a young patient. Diabetes secondary to pancreatic inflammation is a real consideration. Diabetes could be the result of the destruction of β-cells of the pancreas and occurs in up to 60% of patients with chronic calcific pancreatitis. Diabetes is particularly difficult to control as there is concomitant loss of glucagon production.

It should be noted that the gross hypertriglyceridaemia in certain patients with type II diabetes can cause acute pancreatitis but its relationship with chronic pancreatitis is controversial. However, this is far less common than alcohol abuse and cholelithiasis as causes of both acute and chronic pancreatitis.

CT is the initial diagnostic choice for imaging patients with pancreatitis. It is excellent in defining and characterizing the acute, subacute and chronic complications related to both acute and chronic pancreatitis. CT is non-invasive, widely available and quick. This is necessary if the patient is acutely unwell due to severe acute pancreatitis when ultrasound can be difficult. CT is helpful in identifying other causes which may mimic the pain associated with chronic pancreatitis, mainly pancreatitic carcinoma. Patients with chronic pancreatitis are at an increased risk of pancreatitic carcinoma. Evaluation of the pancreas requires a focussed pancreatitic protocol (negative oral contrasts, pre- and triple phase post-contrast studies).

Initially the gland appears normal morphologically and with repeated episodes will lead to irreversible morphological changes. In the early phase of chronic pancreatitis the changes are mild duct dilation with loss of the normal duct tapering, side branch ectasia and subtle wall irregularity of the main duct may be visible on MR imaging. As chronic pancreatitis progresses, there is a spectrum of changes from mildly reduced gland size to advanced uniform fibrous substitution. Calcification will occur by this stage and it is the commonest and most specific CT finding of chronic pancreatitis. Calcification appears as signal void on T1- and T2-weighted MR sequences. The gland may have reduced signal on fat-suppressed non-contrast T1-weighted MR imaging. Contrast in the pancreatic phase will demonstrate reduced and late enhancement of the parenchyma depending on the degree of fibrous replacement. On CT it will result in hypodensity. Subsequent imaging in the venous and late phase will demonstrate high signal on MR and hyperattenuation (bright) on CT of the fibrotic areas. These areas will become more evident and appear more enhanced due to the relative contrast difference if focal areas of fibrosis are adjacent to areas of normal glandular tissue.

References

Etemad B, Whitcomb DC. Chronic pancreatitis: diagnosis, classification and new genetic developments. *Gastroenterology* 2001; **120**: 682–707.

Graziani R, Tapparelli M, Malago R et al. The various imaging aspects of chronic pancreatitis. *Journal of the Pancreas (online)* 2005; **6** (1 Suppl): 73–88.

http://www.emedicine.com/Radio/topic522.htm

Ponette E, Brys P. Plain film. In: *Radiology of the pancreas*, 2nd ed. Berlin: Springer; 1999: 146–7.

Packet 2 Case 5 Question

NEIL COLLIN

Clinical history

A 14-year-old girl presents with painless jaundice. Previously well.

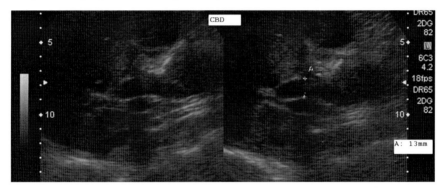

Figure 2.5.1

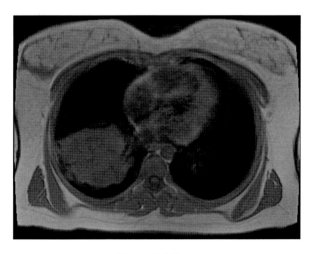

Figure 2.5.2

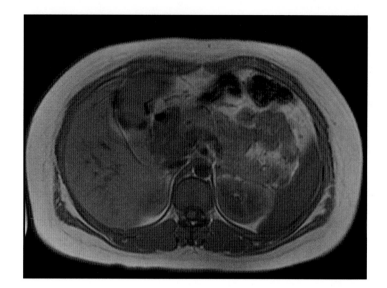

Figure 2.5.3

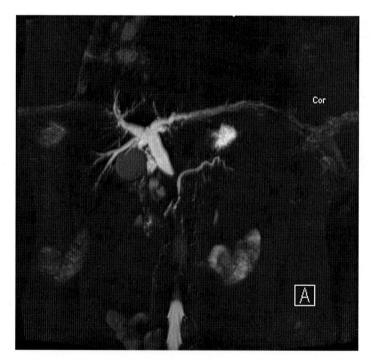

Figure 2.5.4

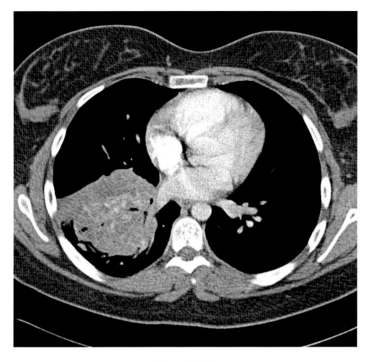

Figure 2.5.5

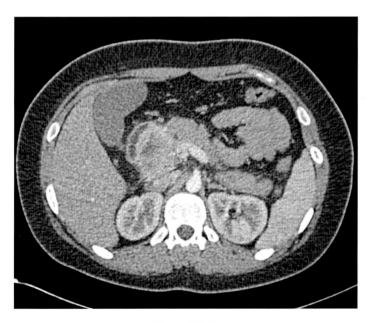

Figure 2.5.6

Packet 2 Case 5 Answer

Model answer

Findings and interpretations

Ultrasound abdomen (Figure 2.5.1)
• Common bile duct is dilated at 13 mm (upper limit of normal is 6 mm).

MRCP (Figure 2.5.4) and MRI abdomen and lower chest (Figures 2.5.2 and 2.5.3)
• Confirms intra- and extrahepatic biliary dilatation.
• No filling defects or calculi seen.
• CBD tapers to complete obstruction in head of pancreas.
• Pancreatic duct not dilated.
• Large abnormal signal mass in head of pancreas and lower lobe of right lung.

CT lower chest/upper abdomen with IV contrast?
• Large obstructing soft tissue mass in head of pancreas.
• Large rounded soft tissue mass with air bronchograms in the lower lobe of the right lung is demonstrated.
• No other abnormality is seen.

Diagnosis

Tumour in right lower lobe of the lung and head of pancreas.

Pancreatic tumours are rare in children; the majority are malignant. Similarly, primary lung tumours are just as rare. The differential diagnosis could either be a primary tumour with metastatic spread or separate synchronous tumours, which is considered unlikely. Another possible differential diagnosis includes lymphoma.

Management

• Urgently refer to paediatric surgical team and paediatric oncology multidisciplinary clinical meeting.
• ERCP to relieve biliary obstruction.
• Percutaneous biopsy (of either lesions) for tissue diagnosis.

In this case

Percutaneous biopsy of the lesion in head of pancreas revealed a primitive neuro-ectodermal tumour. She was referred to a regional paediatric oncology centre and underwent surgical resection and chemoradiotherapy. Tissue biopsy confirmed a primitive neuro ectodermal tumour (Ewing sarcoma family tumour) in the pancreas. This case was thought most likely to be a lung primary tumour with pancreatic metastasis.

Primary pancreatic tumours are rare in childhood, usually malignant and of epithelial origin. Unlike pre-hepatic and intrahepatic causes of jaundice, true obstructive jaundice is very rare in children compared with adults. Accordingly jaundice in the presence of dilated bile ducts should be taken very seriously. Particularly in overweight teenagers, gallstones are the commonest cause. It should be remembered that failure to identify a cause on ultrasound does not definitively exclude either gallstones or other obstructing lesion and should prompt further investigation.

Ewing sarcoma family tumour

Sarcomas are a heterogeneous spectrum of tumours classified according to the tissue they resemble with common histological and immunological features. Ewing's sarcoma (ES) family of tumours consists of Ewing's sarcoma, peripheral neuroectodermal tumour (PNET), Askin tumour (malignant small cell tumour of the thoracopulmonary region) and neuroepithelioma.

The classic Ewing's sarcoma is a small round blue cell tumour and it is the second commonest childhood primary bone cancer after osteosarcoma comprising 10–15% of all bone primaries. It most commonly affects white males in the second decade but can still affect patients in the first and third decade. It is uncommon in the Asian, African and African-American population. Most Ewing's sarcoma occurs in bone, commonly the pelvic bones, femur and tibia. Patients usually present with pain and non-specific symptoms of anorexia, malaise, and low-grade fevers in the more advanced stages. Worrying clinical features are continuing pain and/or night pain especially if there has NOT been any history of trauma.

The more differentiated Ewing's sarcoma encompasses pPNET; peripheral primitive neuroectodermal tumours as in this case. Currently there is no specific immuno-histochemical immune complex that is specific for Ewing's sarcoma and PNET from other undifferentiated tumours. MIC2 is a glycoprotein that is a sensitive marker for the ES/PNET family of tumours. Other neoplasms and even normal tissue can be positive for anti-MIC2. Examples of normal cells that are positive for anti-MIC2 are pancreatic islets, urothelium and sertoli cells. A few examples of neoplastic cell types that are positive for anti-MIC2 are astrocytoma, lymphoma, schwannoma and malignant fibrous histiocytoma. The lung is the commonest extraskeletal site for the ES family of tumours. Diagnosis is made with adequate sampling by open incisional biopsy and should be performed by a specialist orthopaedic oncologist.

Treatment comprises surgical resection to achieve negative margins followed by chemoradiotherapy. Surgery is aimed at preserving limb function if possible.

The five-year survival for patients presenting with metastatic disease is 20–30%. Important prognostic factors are:

• Stage
• primary tumour site
• size
• age
• response to therapy

Diagnostic radiology is highly important in staging and assessment of response to chemotherapy. The following imaging investigations are required – plain films in two orthogonal planes of the entire bone to include the adjacent joints, MRI and/or CT, again to include adjacent joints, and chest CT searching for lung metastases, 99mTc bone scan to search for any other skeletal metastases and FDG-PET, depending on local availability. Metastatic disease is the most important poor prognostic indicator. Patients with isolated pulmonary metastases have an improved prognosis compared with extrapulmonary involvement which has less than 20% survival rate.

References

Alava E, Gerald WL. Molecular biology of the Ewing's sarcoma/primitive neuroectodermal tumor family. *J Clin Oncol* 2000; **18**(1): 204–13.

Bernstein M, Kovar H, Paulussen M et al. Ewing's sarcoma family of tumours: current management. *The Oncologist* 2006; **11**: 503–19.

Grier H. The Ewing family of tumours: Ewing's sarcoma and primitive neuroectodermal tumors. *Paed Clin N Am* 1997; **44**(4): 991–1004.

Takahashi D, Nagayama J, Nagatoshi Y et al. Primary Ewing's sarcoma family tumors of the lung – a case report and review of the literature. *Jap J Clin Oncol* 2007; **37**(11): 874–7.

Packet 2 Case 6 Question

MANDY WILLIAMS

Clinical history

A 58-year-old female became ill whilst on holiday in the Middle East. She presents with fever, confusion and seizure.

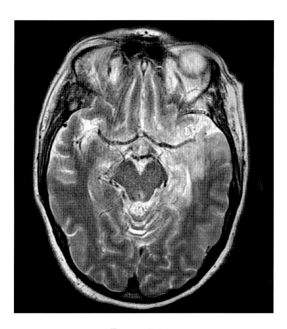

Figure 2.6.1

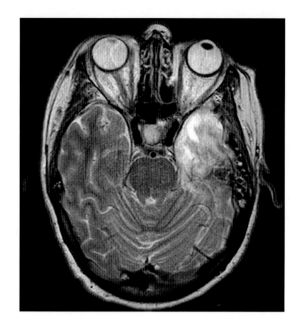

Figure 2.6.2

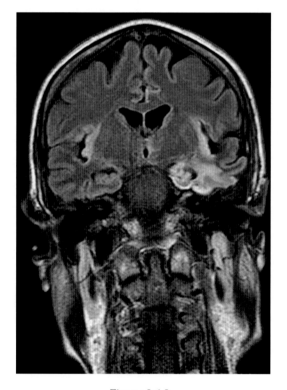

Figure 2.6.3

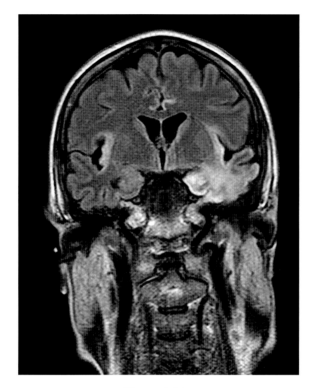

Figure 2.6.4

Packet 2 Case 6 Answer

Model answer

Examination
Non-contrast MRI brain:

- Axial T2-weighted images (Figures 2.6.1 and 2.6.2).
- Coronal FLAIR (fluid attenuated inversion recovery) images (Figures 2.6.3 and 2.6.4).

Observations and interpretations
- There is high signal intensity in both the T2-weighted and FLAIR sequences.
- The high signal is bilateral and located in the temporal lobes especially affecting the hippocampi and more marked on the left.
- The high signal extends along the Sylvian fissures to involve the insular cortex bilaterally.
- There is no mass effect.
- There is no hydrocephalus.
- The affected area involves the limbic system and is bilateral and asymmetrical. The clinical presentation and imaging would point to acute encephalitis.

Diagnosis
Acute herpes simplex virus 1 encephalitis.

Differential diagnosis
Inflammatory causes: meningitis/encephalomeningitis.

Management
The imaging findings need to be relayed immediately to the clinicians so that appropriate antiviral therapy can be started. Without treatment the mortality rate is approximately 40%. With treatment the mortality is about 10%, however a significant number of patients have severe neurological complications.

Herpes simplex virus encephalitis

Herpes simplex virus (HSV) commonly causes oral labial infection. Once an individual is infected, the herpes simplex virus resides in neuronal ganglion. The virus can then enter the central nervous system via the intraneuronal route. HSV is the most common viral agent implicated in encephalitis and accounts for over 90% of cases but it is still a rare disease with an annual incidence of 1–2 per million of the population. HSV encephalitis can be due to primary infection, reinfection (uncommon) or latent reactivation. The clinical manifestation of acute viral encephalitis is fever, headache and altered consciousness. Other less common clinical features are speech disturbances, hemiparesis and seizures. Other viruses include cytomegalovirus (CMV), B virus (cercopithecine herpesvirus), rabies, West Nile virus and Japanese virus (flaviviridae) to name a few.

There are two main subgroups: HSV-1, which typically affects adults and babies over 3 months old, and HSV-2, which affects neonates where there is more diffuse non-focal disease. HSV-1 characteristically involves the temporal lobes and limbic system and will manifest clinically with aphasia, anosmia and temporal lobe seizures. It can involve the frontal lobe, orbital surface and the cingulate gyrus.

HSV-2 usually manifests clinically with subacute symptoms, myelitis or with a strong psychiatric flavour. There are reports of atypical presentations of HSV-2 with brainstem involvement. There are other diseases which can mimic HSV encephalitis: subdural abscess/empyema either due to bacteria, viruses or fungi, tumour and subdural haematomas.

Acyclovir is the treatment of choice for HSV encephalitis. Despite this effective antiviral treatment there is a high morbidity and mortality associated with HSV encephalitis. Relapse can occur after treatment and has been estimated to be as high as 5% but the exact figure is unknown.

Imaging features
These are features in the acute clinical setting.

CT
- Non-contrast CT can be normal particularly early in the clinical course.
- Oedema with gyral effacement particularly affecting the temporal lobes. Intravenous contrast can demonstrate gyriform enhancement.
- Characteristically low attenuation in the temporal lobes. Temporal lobe involvement can either be unilateral or bilateral. The infective process initially starts in one temporal pole and can spread across the midline.
- There may be haemorrhagic change in established cases.

MRI
- T1-weighted imaging reveals low signal intensity in the anterior temporal lobes.
- T2-weighted imaging and FLAIR shows high signal in temporal lobes extending to involve other limbic structures; the insular cortex, amygdala and cingulate gyrus.
- The putamen is spared.
- Haemorrhage: petechial, focal or lobar.
- Diffusion weighting imaging can indicate early change with restricted diffusion in the affected areas.

There are post-complication imaging features affecting the characteristic sites that are demonstrated on CT and MRI which include:

- Encephalomalacia.
- Atrophy.
- Dystrophic calcification.

References

Chu K, Kang DW, Lee JJ, Yoon BW. Atypical brainstem encephalitis caused by herpes simplex virus 2. *Arch Neurol* 2002; **59**: 460–3.

Hui AC, Cheung KF, Liu C et al. Herpes simplex encephalitis in Hong Kong: retrospective review. *Neurol Asia* 2005; **10**: 35–8.

Kimberlin DW. Management of HSV encephalitis in adults and neonates: diagnosis, prognosis and treatment. *Herpes* 2007; **14**(1): 11–16.

Whitley RJ, Gnann JW. Viral encephalitis: familiar infections and emerging pathogens. *Lancet* 2002; **359**: 507–14.

Packet 3 Case 1 Question

OLGA HATSIOPOULOU

Clinical history

A 27-year-old female with dysmenorrhoea and dyspareunia.

Examination

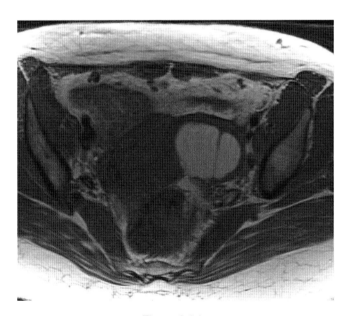

Figure 3.1.1

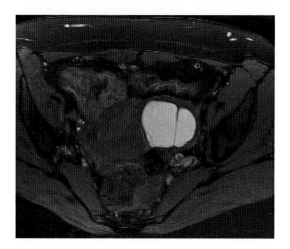

Figure 3.1.2

Answers to follow on page 80

Packet 3 Case 1 Answer

Model answer

Examination
Non-contrast pelvic MRI.

- Axial T1-weighted MR image (Figure 3.1.1).
- Axial T1-weighted MR image with fat saturation (Figure 3.1.2).

Findings and interpretations
- A well-circumscribed septated left adnexal mass adjacent to the uterus and surrounded by ovarian tissue.
- The mass is of high signal intensity on the T1-weighted sequence. The high signal intensity of the lesion persists following fat saturation.
- The lesion causes some mass effect on the uterus with mild deviation of the uterine body to the right. The lesion is unilateral and there is no free fluid in the pelvis.

Diagnosis
Right-sided endometrioma.

The endometrioma appears to be solitary; there are no imaging features to suggest implantation onto peritoneal sites.

Differential diagnosis
In a patient of this age, the differential diagnosis of a solitary high T1-weighted signal ovarian mass includes a haemorrhagic cyst and an ovarian dermoid. In the case of the dermoid, the high T1-weighted signal will be suppressed following fat saturation.

Other possibilities include:

- An ovarian neoplasm, where enhancing nodules and peritoneal deposits may be present.
- A tubo-ovarian abscess where there is a history of infection and stranding of the adjacent soft tissues may be present. This would be helpful in differentiating the lesion from an endometrioma.

Management

Referral to the gynaecological team.

Symptoms can be controlled with gonadotrophin-releasing hormone (GnRH) therapy. Infertility is managed by laparoscopic resection and laser surgery.

Endometriosis

Endometriosis is the presence of functional endometrial tissue outside the endometrium and myometrium. It is a common benign gynaecological condition seen most commonly in women of reproductive age. Endometriosis can occur in teenagers and a small percentage (5%) is seen in post-menopausal women.

Symptoms can be cyclical and hormone dependent with improvement during pregnancy and post menopause.

Patients can be asymptomatic or may present with dysmenorrhoea, dyspareunia, pelvic pain and infertility. Up to 50% of patients with endometriosis are subfertile.

Endometriosis implants can occur anywhere within the peritoneal cavity and can be seen as deposit on the bowel serosa, which can result in cyclical rectal bleeding. Endometriosis is a term that encompasses endometrial deposits/implants, endometrioma and adhesions. There are several theories on the pathophysiology of endometriosis – retrograde menstruation, coelomic metaplasia, and vascular and lymphatic metastasis; however, no single theory explains all the features of the disease process.

The ovary is the most common site of involvement in the form of complex ovarian cysts; endometriomas (chocolate cyst) containing blood products and haemorrhage is usually recurrent. Chocolate cysts are pseudocysts; they do not have a true epithelial lining and are formed by invagination of the ovarian cortex.

Other sites of involvement in endometriosis within the peritoneal cavity are the uterosacral ligaments, posterior broad ligament, the pouch of Douglas, the uterine peritoneal reflection, the fallopian tubes, the rectosigmoid, the urinary tract (most commonly involved is the bladder) and scar tissue. Distant sites are rare and have been reported with deposits in the lungs and the central nervous system.

The initial investigation is ultrasound: transabdominal and transvaginal, transvaginal being more sensitive. Endometriomas on ultrasound have a range of appearance from simple anechoic cysts to low-level echoic cysts. The classic appearance is a homogenous low-level echoic cyst (Figure 3.1.6). They may appear solid, unilocular or multilocular with either thin or thick septations and may contain a fluid–fluid level. There is no intracystic Doppler signal, but there may be perilesional Doppler signal. Lack of intralesional Doppler signal helps differentiate a complex solid- appearing lesion from a malignancy but it cannot exclude the diagnosis and is not specific for an endometrioma. Endometriosis is usually a benign condition but there has been reported risk of ovarian cancer associated with this disease and any demonstration of nodularity or solid-appearing tissue requires further evaluation.

Characteristic MR imaging features of an endometrioma is a homogenously hyperintense T1-weighted lesion that does not suppress with fat saturation (Figures 3.1.1 and 3.1.2). Endometriomas show variable T2-weighted signal, from intermediate (Figures 3.1.3 and 3.1.4) to high signal. Layering of blood products with a fluid–fluid level is a typical finding (Figure 3.1.5), high and low T2-weighted signal. A peripheral rim of low T2-weighted signal may be seen due to chronic blood products. Post contrast, there may be peripheral enhancement of the fibrous wall but the intracystic contents do not enhance.

A characteristic feature is the location of the ovaries in close proximity to each other and the uterus due to adhesions, the 'kissing ovaries' sign, as demonstrated in Figure 3.1.5.

Endometriotic deposits (plaque) can be seen as intermediate signal intensity masses with foci of high T1-weighted signal and low T2-weighted signal masses. A characteristic

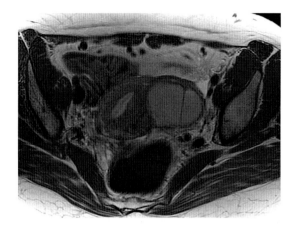

Figure 3.1.3 Axial T2-weighted image.

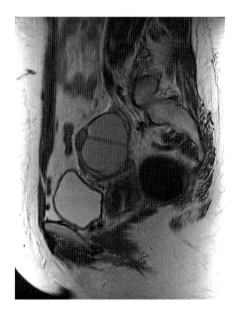

Figure 3.1.4 Sagittal T2-weighted image.

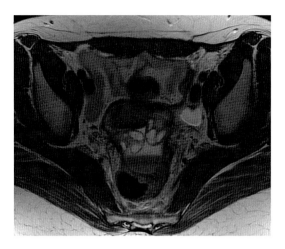

Figure 3.1.5 Axial T2-weighted image.

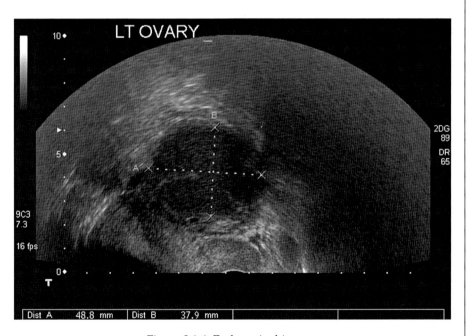

Figure 3.1.6 Endovaginal image.

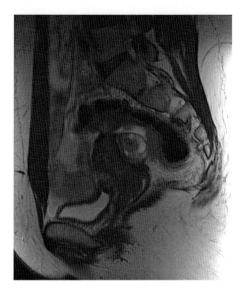

Figure 3.1.7 Sagittal T2-weighted image.

finding of a peritoneal plaque on T2-weighted sequence is that of a low signal intensity mass arising from the dorsal aspect of the uterine body extending to the anterior surface of the sigmoid colon (see Figure 3.1.7). The typical tethering of the bowel and the layering of the ovarian endometrioma is also demonstrated in Figure 3.1.7.

The gold standard for diagnosis is laparoscopy. The deposits are seen as blue-brown, red or black stains, and nodules and scarring will be evident on laparoscopy.

References

Del Frate C, Girometti R, Pittino M et al. Deep retroperitoneal pelvic endometriosis: MR imaging appearance with laparoscopic correlation. *RadioGraphics* 2006; **26**(6): 1705–18.

Hricak H. *Diagnostic imaging: gynecology,* 1st ed. Amirsys/Elsevier; 2007: 7–166, 7–170.

Kinkel K, Frei KA, Balleyguier C, Chapron C. Diagnosis of endometriosis with imaging: a review. *Eur Radiol* 2006; **16**(2): 285–98.

Kocakoc E, Bhatt S, Dogra VS. Endometriosis. *Ultrasound Clin* 2008; **3**: 399–414.

Poder L, Qayyum A, Goldstein RB. Use of MR imaging for further evaluation of sonographically detected adnexal pathology. *Ultrasound Clin* 2006; **1**: 357–83.

Packet 3 Case 2 Question

JOANNA KASZNIA-BROWN

Clinical history

A 52-year-old man presented with a painful right knee. No history of trauma. Previously fit and well.

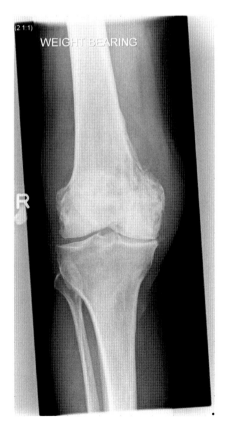

Figure 3.2.1

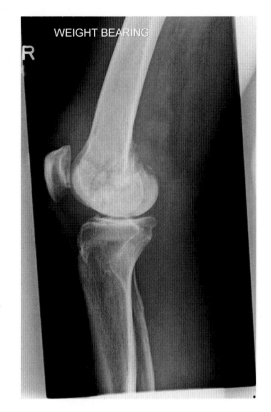

Figure 3.2.2

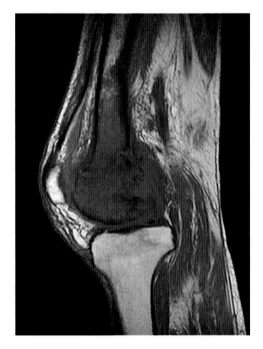

Figure 3.2.3

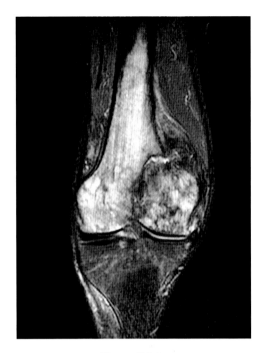

Figure 3.2.4

Packet 3 Case 2 Answer

Model answer

Examination
X-ray right knee – AP and lateral projections (Figures 3.2.1 and 3.2.2).

MRI right knee:
- Sagittal T1-weighted image (Figure 3.2.3)
- Coronal STIR (short tau inversion recovery) image (Figure 3.2.4).

Findings

X-ray
- Ill-defined large lytic lesion with a permeative/moth-eaten appearance in the metaphysis and epiphysis of the right distal femur.
- Destruction of the cortex on the posterior aspect of the metaphysis.
- Periosteal new bone formation.
- Adjacent soft tissue mass, no visible calcifications.

MRI of the right knee
- Large diffuse lesion in the distal right femur associated with small soft tissue mass.
- Extensive cortical destruction.
- Abnormal signal (low T1-weighted signal and high signal on STIR) involving the epiphysis, metaphysis and extends superiorly into the medulla of the diaphysis, which represents an infiltrative process and marrow replacement.
- Oblique fracture through the medial condyle of the right femur.
- Proximal tibia and joint space appear normal.
- No focal fluid collection seen.

Interpretation

- Destructive lytic lesion in the distal right femur with periosteal reaction and a soft tissue mass.
- Extensive bone marrow infiltration.
- Pathological fracture through the medial femoral condyle.

Differential diagnosis

- Metastasis.
- Osteomyelitis.
- Lymphoma.
- Primary bone neoplasm (reticulum cell sarcoma, myeloma, osteosarcoma, Ewing's sarcoma in the younger age group).

Management

- Urgent referral to orthopaedic team if suspicious of primary bone neoplasm – referral to local sarcoma team.
- Bone scan.
- CT chest and abdomen/pelvis with intravenous contrast for staging.
- MRI right femur to assess local spread.
- Biopsy to be performed by the sarcoma team.

In this case

Biopsy of the lesion was performed, which confirmed the diagnosis of primary bone lymphoma.

Primary bone lymphoma

Primary bone lymphoma (PBL), also known as reticulum cell sarcoma or histiocytic lymphoma, is a rare malignant bone neoplasm that accounts for less than 5% of all primary bone tumours. Ninety-five percent of cases are of the non-Hodgkin type.

Primary bone lymphoma can occur at any age, with peak prevalence in the 3rd to 6th decade. Fifty percent of patients are younger than 40 years, but it is very rare in children younger than 10 years of age. It is more common in males (male: female = 2:1). The lower femur (especially the metadiaphysis) is the commonest site of involvement and is affected in 25% of cases. Other sites include upper tibia, humerus, pelvis, ribs and vertebrae. PBL presents with intermittent bone pain, which can persist for months. Other signs include local swelling, a palpable mass with systemic symptoms; weight loss and fever.

The radiographic appearance of PBL has a wide spectrum of findings from normal bone to a diffusely permeative process with cortical destruction and soft tissue involvement. The most common feature is a lytic-destructive pattern with a permeative or moth-eaten appearance. Pathological fractures are commonly found in malignant bone tumours and are found in about 25% of cases.

More specific features common to the round cell tumours (primary bone lymphoma, multiple myeloma and Ewing's sarcoma) include relatively mild cortical destruction and periosteal reaction in the presence of extensive marrow involvement and a surrounding soft tissue mass. These patients usually present with mild pain and are in a good general condition despite the size of the lesion.

Treatment of PLB involves radiation and chemotherapy. Patients with a PLB have the best prognosis compared to other primary bone sarcomas.

References

Heyning FH, Kroon HM, Hogendoorn PC et al. MR imaging characteristics in primary lymphoma of bone with emphasis on non-aggressive appearance. *Skeletal Radiol* 2007; **36**(10): 937–44.

Krishnan A, Shirkhoda A, Tehranzadeh J et al. Primary bone lymphoma: radiographic-MRI imaging correlation. *RadioGraphics* 2003; **23**: 1371–87.

Packet 3 Case 3 Question

MARC WILLIAMS

Clinical history

A 6-year-old boy presents with clumsiness and vomiting.

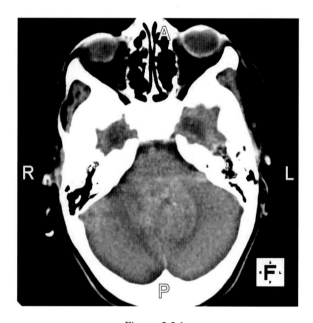

Figure 3.3.1

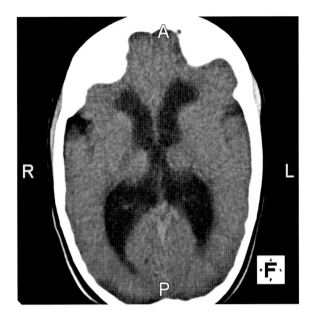

Figure 3.3.2

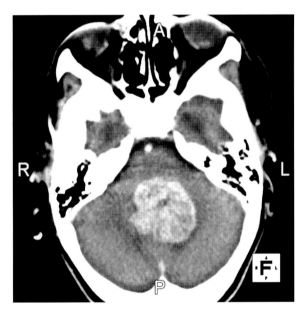

Figure 3.3.3

Packet 3 Case 3 Answer

Clinical history

A 6-year-old boy presents with clumsiness and vomiting.

Model answer

Examination
CT brain pre- (Figures 3.3.1 and 3.3.2) and post-contrast (Figure 3.3.3).

Observations and interpretations
The figures are selected axial images from a CT scan of the brain. Figures 3.3.1 and 3.3.2 are pre-intravenous contrast and Figure 3.3.3 is a post-contrast image. There is a midline mass in the posterior fossa which appears slightly hyperdense to surrounding brain. The mass may contain a tiny area of calcification. There is evidence of hydrocephalus with dilatation of the third and lateral ventricles. The mass demonstrates intense contrast enhancement.

Principal diagnosis and differential diagnosis
The most likely diagnosis is medulloblastoma and the appearances, as described above, are typical for this.
   Differential diagnoses include:

- Cerebellar astrocytoma: this tumour may be cystic, solid or mixed and there may be an enhancing mural nodule. The appearances of this lesion are not typical of this case.
- Ependymoma: this lesion often has calcification and small cystic areas, both of which are less common in medulloblastoma. It may also expand through the foramina of Luschka or Magendie.
- Brainstem glioma: the pons is the commonest location and enhancement is rare.

Management

The patient should be referred urgently to a neurosurgeon for further management.

Medulloblastoma

Approximately 50% of primary brain tumours in children have their origin in the posterior fossa and of these medulloblastoma is the most common primary tumour of the posterior fossa, typically found in males in the 2- to 8-year-old age group. It can arise in adults and is mainly reported in the 20- to 40-year-old age group and rarely beyond 50 years of age. Medulloblastoma is characterized as a primitive neuroectodermal tumour (PNET), usually arising from cells located in the roof of the 4th ventricle. The tumour is highly malignant and has a tendency to seed along cerebrospinal fluid pathways (10–30% of patients demonstrate evidence of this at diagnosis) and may metastasize beyond the central nervous system, usually to bone but liver and lymph nodes are other potential sites for spread.

Associated syndromes include:

- Gorlin syndrome (nevoid basal cell carcinoma syndrome) is an autosomal dominant rare disorder. The syndrome consists of basal cell carcinomas, jaw cysts, palmar and plantar pits, and medulloblastoma. Medulloblastoma in Gorlin syndrome will develop at an earlier age than sporadic causes of medulloblastoma.
- Turcot's syndrome is a genetic disorder consisting of colorectal polyposis and brain tumours. There are two subtypes of hereditary colorectal polyposis: familial adenomatous polyposis (FAP) coli and hereditary non-polyposis colorectal cancer. Medulloblastoma is the most common brain tumour in FAP. Patients with FAP can develop other types of brain tumours: astrocytomas and ependymomas. Hereditary non-polyposis colorectal cancer patients have a tendency for other primary glial tumours – glioblastoma.

Patients with Gorlin and Turcot's syndrome have increased risk of developing secondary malignancies.

Patients usually have only a brief clinical history due to the aggressive nature of the lesion. They usually present with clumsiness, cerebellar signs, blurred vision, papilloedema, dizziness, headache, nausea and vomiting. Seizures are uncommon.

Since medulloblastomas are radiosensitive, treatment is usually a combination of surgery and radiation to the entire neuroaxis. There can be involvement of the leptomeninges in up to 33% at the time of diagnosis. Radiation therapy will have a profound secondary effect on the immature developing neuroaxis with cognitive impairment and growth restriction. There is also a significant increased risk of radiation-induced tumour development as a late complication after radiotherapy. Thus radiation therapy should be limited in patients under the age of 2 years.

Imaging findings of medulloblastoma can be characteristic:

- The tumour tends to be located in the midline of the posterior fossa with a strong predilection for the cerebellar vermis. Since medulloblastomas are highly cellular, they tend to be hyperdense to brain (89%) on non-contrast CT examinations. This helps differentiate medulloblastomas from pilocytic astrocytomas. Heterogeneity due to necrosis and haemorrhage is less commonly seen. There may be surrounding oedema and hydrocephalus occurs in most cases due to obstruction at the level of the fourth ventricle.
- Following intravenous contrast, marked enhancement is evident.
- Calcifications may be seen rarely in the primary tumour unless there has been previous radiation therapy.
- Extension into the subarachnoid space may be demonstrated by the presence of enhancing nodules, particularly in the spinal canal ('drop metastases').
- On MRI, medulloblastomas are low signal on T1-weighted images and can vary from intermediate to high signal on T2-weighted images.
- As is the case on CT, avid enhancement on MRI is characteristic, although a slightly more heterogeneous pattern of enhancement may be seen.

- Areas of calcification are seen as signal voids on MRI and are therefore better seen on CT.
- MRI may demonstrate subarachnoid spread as high signal foci in the subarachnoid space on post-contrast T1-weighted imaging. Midline sagittal imaging of the spine is especially useful in this regard.

The imaging features, in combination with the tumour location and patient age, are able to suggest the diagnosis in many cases.

References

Dahnert W. *Radiology review manual*. Philadelphia: Lippincott, Williams & Wilkins; 2003: 299.

Farrell CJ, Plotkin SR. Genetic causes of brain tumors: neurofibromatosis, tuberous sclerosis, von Hippel-Lindau and other syndromes. *Neurol Clin* 2007; **25**: 925–46.

Koeller KK, Rushing EJ. From the Archives of the AFIP. Medulloblastoma: a comprehensive review with radiologic-pathologic correlation. *RadioGraphics* 2003; **23**: 1613–37.

Medulloblastoma. 12 Apr, 2007. Available at: http://www.emedicine.com/RADIO/topic434.htm

Rowe J. Late neoplastic complications after radiation treatments for benign intracranial tumors. *Neurosurg Clin North Am* 2006; **17**: 181–5.

Packet 3 Case 4 Question

KIAT TAN

Clinical history

A 25-year-old Caucasian presents with a 3-week history of back pain that has significantly deteriorated in the last few days.

(a)   (b)

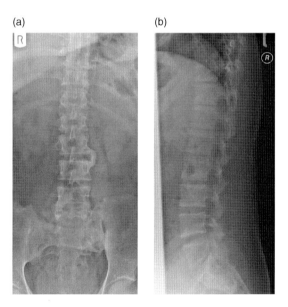

Figure 3.4.1a and b

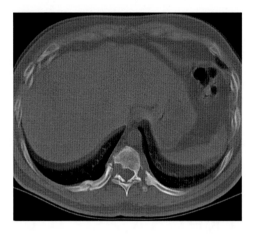

Figure 3.4.2

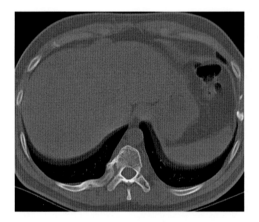

Figure 3.4.3

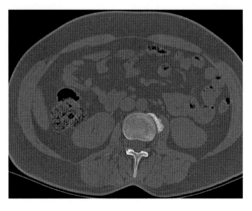

Figure 3.4.4

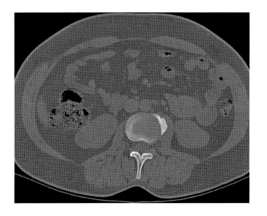

Figure 3.4.5

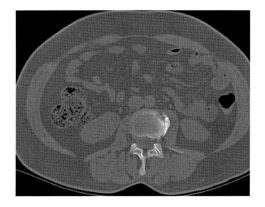

Figure 3.4.6

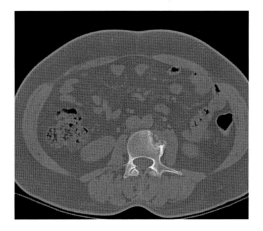

Figure 3.4.7

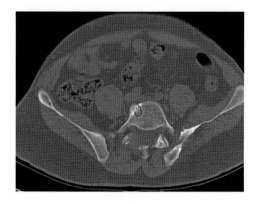

Figure 3.4.8

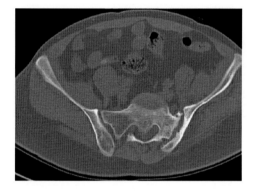

Figure 3.4.9

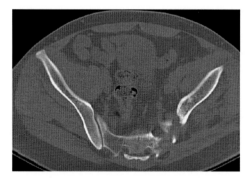

Figure 3.4.10

Answers to follow on page 100

Packet 3 Case 4 Answer

Model answer

Examination
- Plain AP and lateral radiographs of the spine.
- Selected CT images of the spine on bone window.

Findings and interpretations

Plain radiographs
- Destruction of the head of the left 10th rib.
- Some loss of disc height at L2/3.
- Ill definition and possible sclerosis at the end plates at L2/3.
- Ill-defined sclerosis around the left pedicle of L3.
- Calcification just to the left of the L2/3 vertebral body projected over the psoas.
- Disruption of the left sacroiliac joint with superior displacement of the left innominate bone.
- Sclerosis around the left sacroiliac joint.
- Prominent left psoas muscle.

CT scan
- Bony destruction at multiple sites and levels in the rib and vertebral bodies. Some of these are associated with sequestrum and/or new bone formation.
- Gross destruction of the left sacroiliac joint with bony destruction and sclerosis.
- Lens-shaped calcification deep to the psoas muscle.

Diagnosis
Skeletal tuberculosis with psoas muscle abscess.

Differential diagnosis
- Multifocal pyogenic/fungal osteomyelitis.
- Metastatic disease.

Management
(1) Needs urgent referral to the chest physicians.
(2) Bone biopsy is required.

(3) Chest radiograph.
(4) Tuberculin skin testing.

Skeletal tuberculosis

Tuberculosis is an infectious disease caused mainly by *Mycobacterium tuberculosis*. It is very common and according to a World Health Organization estimate approximately one-third of the world's population is currently infected with TB bacilli. It is particularly prevalent in certain regions of the world (sub-Saharan Africa and South-East Asia) and human migration plays a large role in the epidemiology of this infectious disease.

Over the years, TB has become resistant to first-line drug therapy and there has been emergence of multidrug-resistant TB (MDR-TB). MDR-TB is where TB bacilli are resistant to at least two first-line anti-TB drugs (isoniazid and rifampicin). It is treatable but requires up to 2 years of treatment. Even more lethal has been the combination of infection with HIV and TB, which has led to the emergence of extensively drug-resistant TB (XDR-TB). The main impact has been primarily in developing countries where the prevalence of both MTB and HIV infection is high.

Involvement of the skeletal system is uncommon especially in the immunocompetent patient, even in countries where the disease is endemic. Multifocal skeletal tuberculosis occurs as a result of haematogenous spread from the lungs. It can spread directly from adjacent soft tissue structures (discs) or lymphatic spread from infected lymph nodes. Skeletal tuberculosis is seen in up to 2–3% of patients with extra-pulmonary TB. The disease typically involves the spine, sacroiliac joints and weight-bearing joints; however, any bone or joint may be affected.

Vertebral TB, also known as Pott's disease, occurs in 50% of patients with skeletal TB. Involvement of the sacroiliac joint is rare and even rarer is the co-involvement of the spine with very few cases reported in the literature. Clinically the symptoms of skeletal tuberculosis are insidious and non-specific. Pain is most common; sinus drainage, joint swelling and limited motion can occur. Unifocal spinal tuberculosis can be difficult to differentiate from pyogenic infection. However, the chronicity of the disease, presence of new bone formation and soft tissue calcification all point towards a diagnosis of tuberculosis. Skeletal TB is also most often multifocal in nature. In the adult the mid-thoracic region is most commonly involved whilst in the paediatric population it is the cervical spine.

This case illustrates the classical plain radiographic features of spinal/sacroiliac joint TB. The joint space is involved from adjacent epiphyseal bone or haematogenous dissemination. Early synovitis, granulation tissue and effusion develop. Eventually the cartilage is destroyed peripherally initially with preservation of the joint space; bone demineralization and caseation necrosis occurs. In the later stage, there is complete destruction with collapse of the vertebral body. Extensive destruction can result in compromise of the vertebral canal and various neurological syndromes, the most significant being spinal cord compression.

CT is useful in detecting the extent of bony involvement whilst MR imaging is used to assess the extent of any soft tissue complications particularly sinus tract formation and epidural extension. Bone scintigraphy with technetium is useful in the early stages, is more sensitive than CT or plain radiographs and will detect occult multiple sites. Confirmation of TB osteomyelitis requires microbiological confirmation and may require polymerase chain reaction (PCR) if culture or the Ziel Nielsen stain cannot yield the acid-fast bacilli.

A possible differential is metastatic disease but it does not classically cross the end plates of two adjacent vertebral bodies. In addition, the presence of soft tissue calcification is unusual (although it can be seen in osteosarcoma and some adenocarcinomas).

References

De Vuyst D, Vanhoenacker F, Gielen J, Bernaerts A, De Schepper AM. Imaging features of musculoskeletal tuberculosis. *Eur Radiol* 2003; **13**: 1809–19.

Gelel F, Sabah D, Dogan R, Avci A. Multifocal skeletal tuberculosis involving the lumbar spine and a sacroiliac joint: MR imaging findings. *Diagn Interv Radiol* 2006; **12**: 139–41.

Global tuberculosis control report 2008. Available at: http://www.who.int/mediacentre/factsheets/fs104/en/

Marudanaygam A, Gnanadoss JJ. Multifocal skeletal tuberculosis: a report of three cases. *The Iowa Orthopaedic Journal* 2006; **26**: 151–3.

Teo EL, Peh WC. Imaging of tuberculosis of the spine. *Singapore Med J* 2004; **45**: 439–44.

Packet 3 Case 5 Question

NEIL COLLIN

Clinical history

A 25-year-old female presents with left loin to groin pain.

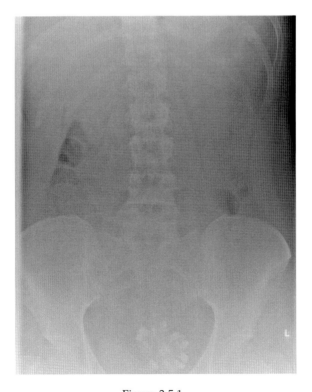

Figure 3.5.1

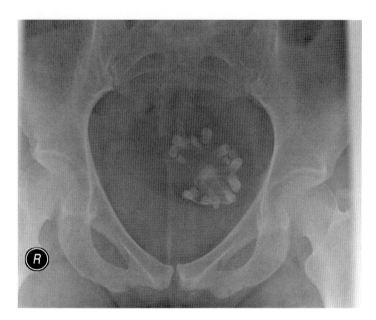

Figure 3.5.2

Answers to follow on page 106

Packet 3 Case 5 Answer

Model answer

Examination
Frontal radiographs of the abdomen and pelvis.

Findings and interpretation
Abdominal radiograph:

- 10 cm well-defined fat density lesion is projected over the mid pelvis.
- Multiple dense calcifications centrally with dental morphology (well-defined crowns and roots) are seen.
- There are more amorphous areas of calcification/ossification adjacent to dental structures seen.
- Bowel gas pattern appears normal.
- No renal tract calcification is demonstrated; the renal outlines and psoas shadows appear normal.
- No bony abnormality.

Diagnosis
Ovarian dermoid.
The presentation with pain may imply torsion/infarction or may relate to another pathology.
Malignant germ cell tumour less likely in this age group.

Management
- Referral to gynaecology for laparoscopy/excision.
- Ultrasound pelvis to assess ovaries.
- If clinical history, urine dipstick testing, etc. suggestive of other pathology such as renal colic.
- CT may be helpful.

In this case
The patient was referred to gynaecology and underwent laparoscopic resection. Histology confirmed a benign ovarian dermoid. It did not appear to have twisted or bled and the cause of pain was unclear.

Ovarian dermoid

Mature teratoma is a true hamartoma and is otherwise known as a dermoid cyst. They are the most common benign ovarian tumours in females less than 45 years of age. It contains mature cell lines in an abnormal location and is thought to result from abnormal development of a primary oocyte and can include tissue from two or more embryonic germ cell layers. Contents include fat, hair, neural tissue, bone and teeth, in varying degrees of differentiation.

They are almost always benign. Rarely, malignant transformation can occur, typically to invasive squamous cell carcinoma. Any of the cell lines can theoretically undergo malignant transformation. There are case reports of melanoma arising in an ovarian dermoid. In older age groups, malignant germ cell tumours can have a similar appearance. Other malignant ovarian tumours can contain fat or calcification, although the presence of such well-differentiated tissue is rare.

Ovarian dermoids tend to be slow-growing tumours and are often asymptomatic. Typically they are small (2–5 cm) at presentation but can become very large (in excess of 20 cm). They can present with pain or pressure symptoms, or when a complication occurs. Torsion is the most common complication, followed by bleeding. Rupture with possible chemical peritonitis and subsequent granulomatous peritoneal deposits are also described.

Treatment usually involves laparoscopic resection; however, larger dermoids may require an open surgical approach if there is a considered risk of rupture and spillage of contents causing chemical peritonitis. The rationale for removal revolves around the real risk of torsion or bleeding and the more theoretical risk of malignant transformation. Given the multitude of cell types within dermoid tumours and risk of rupture, biopsy is not a viable option. Another surgical consideration is minimizing adhesions as the majority of patients are still in their reproductive years. If there are any concerns about the possibility of a malignant ovarian cyst, then open surgical approach is required.

They demonstrate a broad range of findings on imaging due to the varying degree of tumour content. Dermoids may contain an echogenic tubercle, seen on ultrasound and known as a Rokitansky nodule. If bone and teeth are present, as in this illustrated case, they tend to be located in this nodule. Ultrasound findings follow the basic principle of tissue or fluid echogenicity depending on the content of the lesion. Hair is seen as echogenic bands.

The demonstration of fat within a cyst, with or without thin rim of wall calcification, is highly suggestive of a mature teratoma on CT.

MR imaging is a useful adjunct in assessment of ultrasound indeterminate lesions.

On MR the sebaceous component will have a high signal on T1- and T2-weighted sequences due to the fat content, but T2 signal can be more variable in signal intensity. Fat suppression techniques will help differentiate fat from haemorrhage with lesions that are high on T1-weighted sequences.

Teeth or bone will be low signal on all sequences. If there is any suspicion of malignant transformation or doubt about the diagnosis, post-contrast MR is useful to assess any solid components which will enhance.

References

Berg C, Berndorff U, Diedrich K, Malik E. Laparoscopic management of ovarian dermoid cysts: a series of 83 cases. *Arch Gynaecol Obstet* 2002; **266**(3): 126–9.

Jung SE, Lee JM, Rha SE et al. CT and MR imaging of ovarian tumors with emphasis on differential diagnosis. *RadioGraphics* 2002; **22**: 1306–25.

Mironov S, Akin O, Pandit-Taskar N, Hann LE. Ovarian cancer. *Radiol Clin N Am* 2007; **45**: 149–66.

Schwartz RA. *Dermoid cyst.* June 2007. Available at: http://www.emedicine.com/derm/TOPIC686.HTM

Shawki O, Ramadan A, Askalany A, Bahnassi A. Laparoscopic management of ovarian dermoid cysts: potential fear of dermoid spill, myths and facts. *Gynecol Surg* 2007; **4**: 255–60.

Packet 3 Case 6 Question

INDRAN DAVAGNANAM

History

A 24-year-old male presents with neck pain and dysphasia.

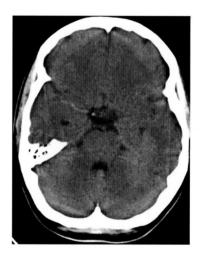

Figure 3.6.1

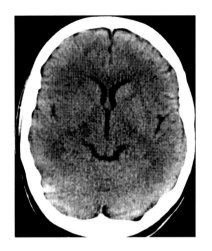

Figure 3.6.2

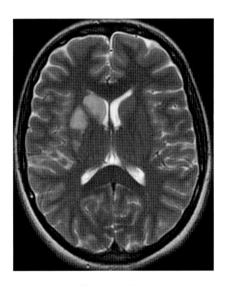

Figure 3.6.3

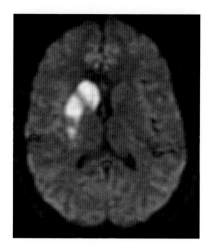

Figure 3.6.4

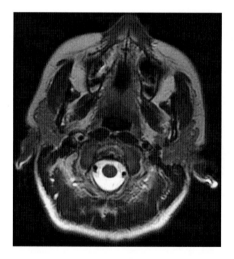

Figure 3.6.5

Answers to follow on page 112

Packet 3 Case 6 Answer

Model answer

Examination
Unenhanced CT and MRI brain examinations.

Findings
- Unenhanced CT of the brain with a hyperdense right middle cerebral artery (MCA) (Figure 3.6.1).
- Unenhanced CT of the brain demonstrating subtle but perceptible low density of the right head of caudate and lentiform nuclei (Figure 3.6.2).
- Axial T2-weighted image with hyperintensity of the right head of caudate and lentiform nuclei (Figure 3.6.3).
- DWI (B = 1000) image demonstrating hyperintensity in the same regions (Figure 3.6.4).
- Axial T2-weighted image with asymmetrical apparent reduction in calibre of the right petrous internal carotid artery (ICA), with surrounding crescentic hyperintensity (Figure 3.6.5).

Interpretations
- Right MCA thrombus (dense MCA sign).
- Hyperacute/acute right MCA territory infarct (lenticulostriate artery territory).
- Right ICA dissection.

Diagnosis
Right ICA dissection causing a right MCA territory infarct.

Management
- Contact the clinicians/stroke team for anticoagulation and subsequent rehabilitation management depending on functional deficit.
- Further imaging of the carotids – ultrasonography (US), CT angiography or contrast-enhanced MR angiography (CEMRA).

Carotid artery dissection and stroke in young adults

Stroke presents clinically with a sudden onset of neurological deficit. It is very common especially in the elderly population with the incidence of stroke increasing with age. Approximately 80% of strokes are caused by cerebral ischaemia due to arterial occlusion and the remaining 20% is due to haemorrhage. Other causes in the younger population (younger than 50 years) should be sought, as atherosclerotic disease risk is highly unlikely to be the cause in this age group. According to the literature, approximately 20% of strokes in younger patients are due to cervicocerebral arterial dissection and 80% are secondary to extracranial internal carotid artery dissection.

Arterial dissection should always be suspected in young adults acutely presenting with a large cerebral arterial infarction. This may present clinically distinct as either anterior or posterior circulation infarcts representing internal carotid and vertebral artery dissections respectively. Other clinical syndromes are recognized depending on the location; pain, headache, partial Horner's syndrome (sympathethic fibres course along the internal carotid artery) and lower cranial palsies.

Carotid dissections unlike atherosclerotic disease typically spare the carotid bulb and occur distal to the bifurcation. A history of trauma (which may range from mild to severe) is most common but conditions such as fibromuscular dysplasia and collagen vascular diseases such as Ehlers-Danlos (autosomal dominant) or Marfan's syndrome predisposed to dissection may be found, although uncommon. Other conditions that have an increased risk of carotid dissection are alpha-1 anti-trypsin deficiency and hyperhomocysteinaemia, which have been recently reported along with more common vascular risk factors such as smoking and hypertension.

Cross-sectional imaging aims to confirm the presence of a hyperacute/acute stroke (restricted diffusion: high signal on diffusion weighted imaging and corresponding low signal on the apparent diffusion coefficient map) and evidence of a dissection. This may be seen as a dissection flap or altered blood products within the false lumen on CT angiography (CTA), MRI/MRA or ultrasound. There are several MR angiography (MRA) techniques available: time of flight (2D or 3D) and phase contrast. On MRI, dual-echo and standard T1-weighted imaging demonstrates a variable crescentic area of hyperintensity (crescent sign), while on CT a cuff of soft-tissue 'thickening' is sometimes apparent. Fat suppression can be also helpful on MRI to differentiate the thrombus from surrounding soft tissues. Signal void is demonstrated on time of flight. Vessel calibre narrowing is evident on all three modalities especially on contrast-enhanced CTA or MRA. MRA can be used for follow-up imaging especially since repeated CTs will have a significant radiation burden for this younger age group.

Digital subtraction angiography (DSA) is still the gold standard; the imaging features may include irregular vessel narrowing, tapered vessel or complete vessel occlusion.

Acute arterial dissection resulting in stroke is at present a relative contraindication for thrombolysis. Currently management includes the use of heparin/low-molecular-weight heparin and/or anti-platelet agents (aspirin or clopidogrel) to prevent further thrombus formation, propagation and embolization. Recanalization does not occur after complete occlusion of the vessel. Surgery and acute endovascular treatment currently has a limited role in management of dissections. Any associated subarachnoid haemorrhage, which may occur with intracranial dissection disease, is an indication for surgical intervention.

References

Atlas SW. *Magnetic resonance imaging of the brain and spine*, Vol I, 4th edn. Lippincott, Williams & Wilkins; 2008: 851–3.

Flis CM, Jäger HR, Sidhu PS. Carotid and vertebral artery dissections: clinical aspects, imaging features and endovascular treatment. *Eur Radiol* 2007; **17**(3): 820–34.

Klufas RA, Hsu L, Barnes PD, Patel MR, Schwartz RB. Dissection of the carotid and vertebral arteries: imaging with MR angiography. *AJR* 1995; **164**: 673–7.

Osborn AG, Blaser S, Salzman K et al. *Diagnostic imaging: brain,* 1st ed. Amirsys/ Elsevier; 2004: 28–31, 76–79.

Thanvi B, Munshi SK, Dawson SL, Robinson TG. Carotid and vertebral artery dissection syndromes. *Postgrad Med J* 2005; **81**: 383–8.

Packet 4 Case 1 Question

MONICA KHANNA

Clinical history

A 76-year-old male presents with a buttock mass and lower abdominal pain.

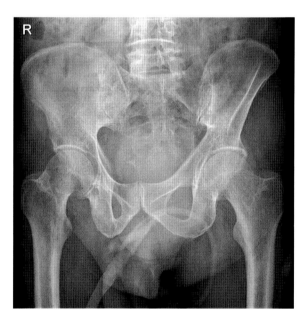

Figure 4.1.1

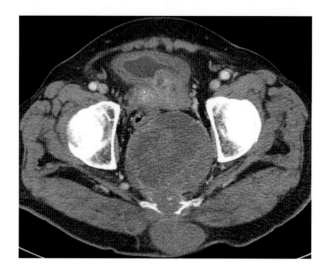

Figure 4.1.2

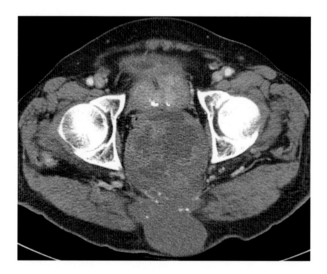

Figure 4.1.3

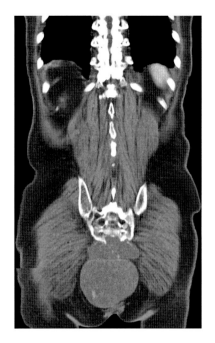

Figure 4.1.4

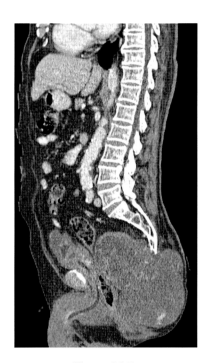

Figure 4.1.5

Packet 4 Case 1 Answer

Model answer

Examination
- Pelvic AP film (Figure 4.1.1).
- Axial enhanced CT pelvis (Figures 4.1.2 and 4.1.3).
- Coronal enhanced CT pelvis (Figure 4.1.4).
- Sagittal enhanced CT pelvis (Figure 4.1.5).

Findings and interpretations

- Pelvic AP radiograph. There is a soft tissue density projected over the distal sacrum causing bony destruction. The lesion extends inferiorly below the level of the pubic rami.
- Axial, coronal and sagittal enhanced CT pelvic images. There is a large soft tissue mass centred at the lower sacrum and coccyx with anterior and posterior extraosseous extension. Bony destruction of the underlying distal sacrum and coccyx is demonstrated. The lesion demonstrates some enhancement and small foci of calcification. The rectum is displaced anterolaterally. The bladder wall is thickened.

Diagnosis
Chordoma.

Differential diagnosis
An expansile lesion of the sacrum could also include:

- Giant cell tumour
- Chondrosarcoma
- Ependymoma
- Plasmocytoma
- Solitary metastatic deposit.

However, calcification on CT, origin at the sacrococcygeal junction and the presence of internal septations are features that distinguish chordoma from other sacral neoplasms.

Management

- Further evaluation with an MRI to include the clivus and skull base, CT chest and bone scan.
- Urgent surgical referral to the bone and soft tissue tumour unit.

Further management is assessment for biopsy and surgical excision.

Chordoma

Chordomas are rare primary bone tumours. They are histologically low-grade, usually initially do not metastasize but are locally aggressive. Two to four percent of all primary spinal tumours are chordomas. They are the most common primary malignant sacral tumour and arise from notochordal remnants most commonly in the midline or a paramedian location. They usually arise in the vertebral body and occur most commonly between the ages of 40 and 70 being twice as common in men. These tumours can occur in the paediatric population but are uncommon. They can be found throughout the axial skeleton with a predilection for the sacrococcygeal (50–60%) or clival regions (35%). The order of distribution in the mobile spine is cervical > lumbar > thoracic. In the cervical region, C2 is most commonly involved.

Signs and symptoms of primary bone tumours include nocturnal pain, pathological fractures and in particular chordoma may present with myelopathy or cranial nerve symptoms. Due to their slow growth sacrococcygeal chordomas may enlarge, cause compression and displacement on the rectum and present with constipation.

Chordoma in the sacrococcygeal usually occur in the S4–5 regions. A destructive calcified soft tissue mass seen arising from S4 or S5 is strongly suggestive of a sacrococcygeal chordoma. Usually large and destructive at presentation and can extend anteriorly, laterally and posteriorly. It typically will displace the rectum anteriorly and usually does not invade the pelvic structures due to limitation by the presacral fascia. The lesion may demonstrate matrix calcification on plain radiography; however, plain radiography is not sufficiently sensitive to detect early small lesions.

Rarely dedifferentiated and sarcomatoid components are identified histologically; this is associated with a poor prognosis due to early widespread secondary deposits. Other poor prognostic factors include large size, necrosis on histology and incomplete resection.

These tumours respond poorly to standard radiotherapy unless high doses are used leading to significant collateral damage even with tight field margins. As such, they are treated with surgical resection. On pathological review if there is residual disease on histology, recurrence or palliation, the treatment options include high-energy photon or photon beam radiation with debulking surgery.

Imaging

CT findings

The usual appearance is of a large destructive lesion with a large soft tissue component. Intratumoural calcification is seen in 30–70% of cases.

In contrast to most other spinal bone tumours, chordomas in the spine infiltrate the disc spaces as they spread to involve other vertebral bodies.

MR findings

The tumour typically forms a well-defined encapsulated multilobulated mass which is of low/intermediate signal on T1-weighted and heterogeneous high signal on T2-weighted/STIR sequenences compared to muscle. It may contain foci of hyperintensity because of haemorrhage and may also have a variable enhancement pattern. On T2-weighted imaging it can have a hypointense rim and multiple internal septae.

Intratumoural calcification will demonstrate low signal on gradient echo and can be substantiated if there is corresponding CT imaging available.

The patient will require full local and distant staging and other imaging investigations will be required: CT chest, abdomen and pelvis. A bone scan may also be required. Tissue diagnosis is necessary for planning of surgical management and any adjuvant therapy. En bloc spondylectomy is a well-recognized surgical treatment option and the goal of surgery is to obtain a clear tumour resection margin. Tissue sampling should be performed by the bone and soft tissue tumour unit as tumour can re-occur along the biopsy tract.

References

Chi JH, Byon A, Hsieh P et al. Epidemiology and demographics for primary vertebral tumors. *Neurosurg Clin N Am* 2008; **19**: 1–4.

Chi JH, Sciubba DM, Rhines L et al. Surgery for primary vertebral tumours: en bloc versus intralesional resection. *Neurosurg Clin N Am* 2008; **19**: 111–17.

Saifuddin A. *Musculoskeletal MRI*. London: Hodder Arnold; 2008.

Sciubba DM, Chi JH. Chordoma of the spinal column. *Neurosurg Clin N Am* 2008; **19**: 5–15.

Soo MYS, Wong L. Sacrococcygeal chordoma, pictorial essay. *J HK Coll Radiol* 2002; **5**: 117–25.

Varga PP, Bors I, Lazary A. Sacral tumors and management. *Orthop Clin N Am* 2009; **40**: 105–23.

Packet 4 Case 2 Question

JOANNA KASZNIA-BROWN

Clinical history

A 56-year-old woman with a 3-week history of worsening lower chest pain on the right side. Past medical history of breast cancer 4 years ago, treated with right mastectomy and axillary clearance. Otherwise, fit and well.

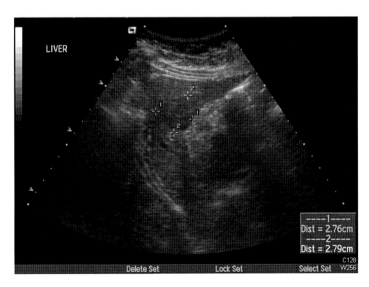

Figure 4.2.1

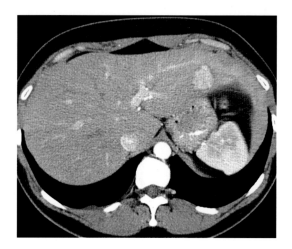

Figure 4.2.2

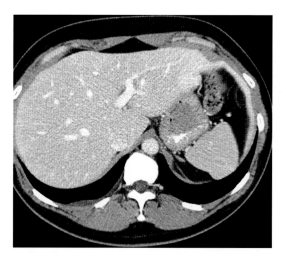

Figure 4.2.3

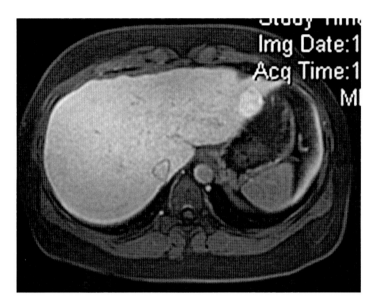

Figure 4.2.4

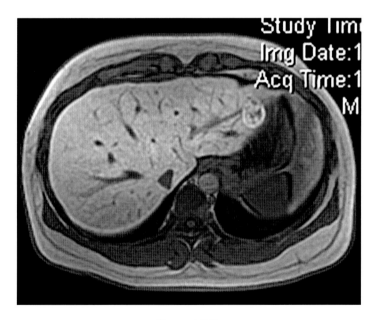

Figure 4.2.5

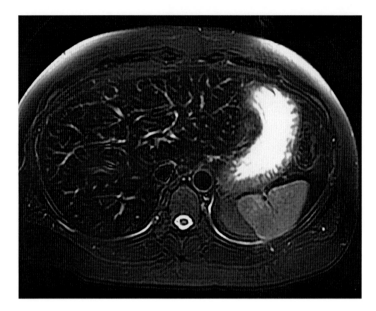

Figure 4.2.6

Answers to follow on page 126

Packet 4 Case 2 Answer

Model answer

Examination
- Ultrasound of the liver (Figure 4.2.1)
- CT liver with intravenous contrast:
  - arterial phase (Figure 4.2.2)
  - porto-venous phase (Figure 4.2.3)
- MRI liver:
  - Axial T1-weighted with gadolinium in the arterial phase (Figure 4.2.4)
  - Axial T1-weighted with gadolinium in porto-venous phase (Figure 4.2.5)
  - Axial T2-weighted with superparamagnetic iron oxide (SPIO) (Figure 4.2.6)

Findings

Ultrasound
There is a homogeneous lesion of decreased echogenicity in the left lobe of the liver, measuring 27×28 mm.

CT
- 2.7 cm well-defined lesion in segment II of the left lobe of the liver.
- Marked vascular enhancement in the arterial phase.
- Similar to background parenchyma in the porto-venous phase.
- No other focal hepatic lesions seen.
- Liver is normal in size, shape and echotexture – no evidence of cirrhosis.
- No pleural effusion or lymphadenopathy seen.

MRI
- Normal general appearance of the liver.
- Well-defined lesion in left lobe of liver with an intense enhancement in arterial phase.
- Washout of contrast in porto-venous phase with a hypointense central scar.
- Loss of signal following iron oxide injection.

Interpretation
Well-defined lesion in left lobe of liver with central scar, intense arterial enhancement and washout in porto-venous phase.

Diagnosis

Focal nodular hyperplasia (FNH).

Differential diagnosis

- Adenoma
- Hepatocellular carcinoma
- Hypervascular metastasis
- Haemangioma

Management

Referral to surgical/gastroenterology team.

Focal nodular hyperplasia

Focal nodular hyperplasia (FNH) is the second most common benign tumour of the liver and is present in 3–8% of the adult population. It is twice as common as hepatocellular carcinoma and is commonly seen in young to middle-aged women (peak age 3rd to 4th decade, M:F = 1:8). It may be associated with hepatic haemangioma (in 23%), meningioma, astrocytoma and arterial dysplasia in other organs.

FNH is not a true neoplasm, but a focal hyperplastic response of hepatocytes to a congenital vascular anomaly. It has no true capsule, but frequently contains a central fibrous scar. It is composed of multiple aggregates of hepatocytes (often containing increased amount of fat, triglycerides and glycogen), Kupffer cells, bile duct proliferation within fibrous septa, but without connection to the biliary tree, and thick-walled arteries radiating from the centre towards the periphery. Portal triads and central veins are absent.

The structure makes it very difficult to differentiate FNH from regenerative nodules in cirrhotic liver and hepatocellular adenoma.

Focal nodular hyperplasia is usually asymptomatic and in 50–90% of patients is an incidental finding. Vague abdominal pain is present in about 10–15% of cases. Oral contraceptives do not cause FNH, but have a trophic effect on its growth.

Focal nodular hyperplasia (FNH) is a well-defined, solitary (in 80–95%) lesion of size less than 5 cm (85%) in an otherwise normal liver. It is seen more often in the right lobe (right:left lobe = 2:1) and close to the liver surface. Calcification is extremely rare.

Differential diagnosis of FNH includes: hepatic adenoma, hepatocellular carcinoma, giant cavernous haemangioma, fibrolamellar carcinoma, hypervascular metastasis and intrahepatic cholangiocarcinoma.

On ultrasound FNH can present as a hypo-, iso- or hyperechoic (33%) homogeneous mass. A hyperechoic central scar is visible in less than 20% of cases.

On an unenhanced CT scan it is a hypo- or isoattenuating homogeneous mass, with a characteristic enhancement pattern after injection of intravenous contrast.

Dense enhancement is seen in the arterial phase, and the lesion becomes iso- to hypodense during the portal venous phase, and isodense on delayed images. Late and prolonged enhancement of the central stellate scar occasionally occurs (delayed washout of contrast from myxomatous scar tissue).

Normal uptake on the sulphur colloid scan seen in 50–70% of cases is almost pathognomonic for FNH. Only FNH contains a sufficient number of Kupffer cells to cause normal or increased uptake.

In 94–100% of patients, the FNH lesion is isointense to hypointense on T1-weighted images. In 6%, the signal intensity on T1-weighted images may be hyperintense; and on T2-weighted images, the lesion is slightly hyperintense to isointense in 94–100% of patients.

The central scar of FNH is hypointense on T1-weighted images, but on T2-weighted images, the central scar shows a variable signal-intensity pattern.

On T2-weighted images, the scar appears hyperintense in 75% of patients and hypointense in 25% of patients.

After the administration of a gadolinium-based contrast agent, the enhancement pattern parallels that of contrast-enhanced CT.

MRI findings are not pathognomonic for FNH, but the use of MRI reticuloendothelial agents, such as superparamagnetic iron oxide (SPIO) and ultrasmall superparamagnetic iron oxide (USPIO), increases the specificity.

On SPIO-enhanced T2-weighted images, FNH shows decreased signal intensity because of iron uptake by Kupffer cells. This finding is not specific to FNH, because hepatocellular adenoma and hepatocellular carcinoma may also contain Kupffer cells.

References

Brancatelli G, Federle MP, Grazioli L et al. Focal nodular hyperplasia: CT findings with emphasis on multiphasic helical CT in 78 patients. *Radiology* 2001; **219**: 61–8.

Dahnert W. *Radiology review manual*, 5th ed. Philadelphia: Lippincott, Williams & Wilkins; 2003: 703–4.

Ferlicot S, Kobeiter H, Van Nhieu JT et al. MRI of atypical focal nodular hyperplasia of the liver: radiology-pathology correlation. *AJR* 2004; **182**: 1227–31.

Mortele KJ, Praet M, Van Vlierberghe, Kunnen M, Ros PR. CT and MR imaging findings in focal nodular hyperplasia of the liver: radiologic–pathologic correlation. *AJR* 2000; **175**: 687–92.

Ruppert-Kohlmayr AJ, Uggowitzer MM, Kugler C et al. Focal nodular hyperplasia and hepatocellular adenoma of the liver: differentiation with multiphasic helical CT. *AJR* 2001; **176**: 1493–8.

Packet 4 Case 3 Question

KATE TAYLOR-ROBINSON

Clinical history

A 10-year-old boy presents with a limp and left-sided hip pain.

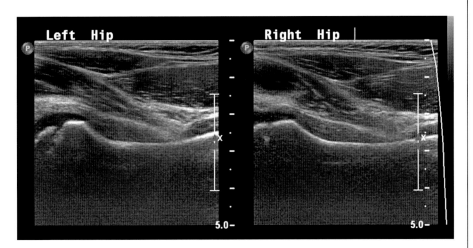

Figure 4.3.1

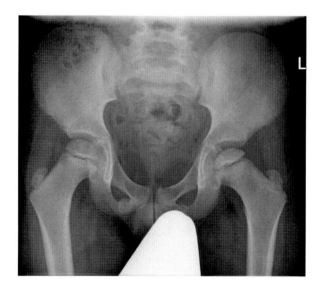

Figure 4.3.2

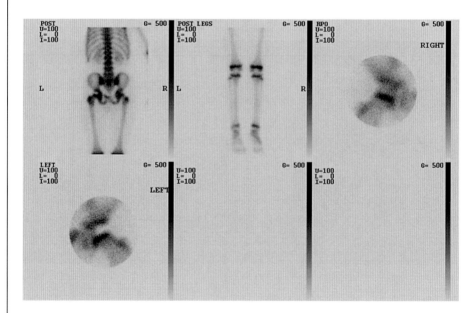

Figure 4.3.3

Answers to follow on page 132

Packet 4 Case 3 Answer

Model answer

Examination
- Ultrasound of the hips (Figure 4.3.1).
- Plain radiograph: AP pelvis (Figure 4.3.2).
- Skeletal scintigraphy – 99mTc MDP bone scan (Figure 4.3.3).

Observations and interpretations
- Ultrasound shows a normal longitudinal anterior view of the femoral head and neck on both sides. In this case there is no evidence of a joint effusion.
- The plain film shows abnormality of the proximal left femoral epiphysis. It is reduced in height, slightly sclerotic and irregular with subtle subchondral lucency. There is inferomedial widening of the joint space but no acetabular changes.
- There is no evidence of slipped femoral epiphysis.
- The bone scan shows a focal photopenic area in the left proximal femoral epiphysis.

Diagnosis
Early stage Legg-Calve-Perthes disease (idiopathic avascular necrosis of the proximal femoral epiphysis).

Differential diagnosis
Osteonecrosis of the proximal femoral epiphysis (avascular necrosis) can be due to other disorders/causes:

- Metabolic: renal disease, steroids (iatrogenic, Cushing's disorders)
- Trauma
- Haemoglobinopathies: Sickle cell, thalassaemia
- Hypercoagulable states: leukaemia, lymphoma
- Post-surgical
- Storage disorders: Gaucher's disease.

Epiphyseal dysplasias could give rise to similar plain film appearances.
Other causes of paediatric hip pain are excluded by this imaging.

Management

Ensure that the paediatric orthopaedic team knows the patient for appropriate management and follow-up.

Legg-Calve-Perthes disease

Legg-Calve-Perthes disease (LCPD) is idiopathic avascular necrosis, or osteochondrosis, of the immature proximal femoral epiphysis. The current consensus hypothesis of the underlying aetiology is hypovascularity due to repetitive vascular insult.

It affects approximately 1:20 000 and is more common in boys (M:F = 5:1). The age range is 3–12 years with a peak around 7 years. In 5–10% it can be bilateral but this is usually asynchronous, so with caution the asymptomatic side can be used as a reference for normal.

The condition usually presents with a painless limp and may later develop hip pain. The child can also present with a painful hip or knee pain and limitation of movement on examination.

Early features can be subtle on plain films and the lateral views of both hips may show the changes more evidently then the AP projection.

Plain radiograph features to look for are sclerotic lines, femoral head depressions, crescent signs and acetabular flattening.

Subtle joint effusions are an early finding, which can be detected by ultrasound.

Both bone scintigraphy and MRI can be used to characterize the changes in early cases since they are more sensitive.

MRI is not only more sensitive than plain radiography, but the imaging technique also lends itself to providing anatomical detail of both ossified and non-ossified structures of the paediatric hip joint without the risk of ionizing radiation. It is also of value in assessing disease progression and for management decisions.

All three orthogonal planes are of value and complementary: the coronal plane allows comparison to the other joint whether it is involved or uninvolved, the sagittal plane allows a better assessment of necrotic bone and the axial plane is useful for assessing the surrounding tissues and structures.

Some of the features you may see on MRI are:

- T1-weighted sequences which demonstrate subchondral fractures as low linear signal changes.
- T2-weighted sequences which can easily depict bright fluid signal either as joint effusions or fluid in the fracture line.
- Necrotic bone which is usually dark on all sequences.

Novel imaging techniques such as dynamic post-contrast MR perfusion and diffusion imaging are being investigated and used in some centres but this is not widely practised.

Bone scintigraphy will show an initial reduction in tracer uptake in the epiphysis followed later by an increase in uptake, which follows the natural history of the condition. The corresponding radiographs show the initial sclerosis and flattening, followed by more painful fragmentation and subchondral fracture, then a remodelling stage with replacement by normal bone. Despite normal bone replacement, the normal growth pattern is disturbed leading to altered morphology. A coxa magna develops; this refers to the typical broad mushroom-shaped epiphysis with a broad shortened metaphysis and corresponding irregular acetabulum.

Treatment is aimed at reducing pressure on the remodelling hip to allow the final joint to be as congruent as possible. Treatment options are either surgical (osteotomy) or non-surgical where the child is treated with bracing.

The earlier the age of onset of disease, the greater the chance of successful congruent remodelling and the lower the risk of premature osteoarthritis. Children older than 8 years have a worse prognosis than their younger counterparts.

Other common causes of paediatric hip pain include:

- Trauma
- Inflammatory: transient synovitis (younger child with effusion) is a common benign self-limiting condition
- Infectious: septic arthritis (usually toxic child with an effusion, hip aspiration is the gold standard in diagnosis, allowing culture and sensitivity for the most appropriate antibiotic regime)
- Slipped proximal femoral epiphysis (characteristic on normal plain film and usually increased uptake on bone scan unless there is associated AVN).

References

Dwek JR. The hip: MR imaging of uniquely pediatric disorders. *Magn Reson Imaging Clin N Am* 2009; **17**: 509–20.

Frick SL. Evaluation of the child who has hip pain. *Orthop Clin N Am* 2006; **37**: 133–40.

Jones LC, Hungerford MW. Outcome measures for evaluation of treatments for osteonecrosis. *Orthop Clin N Am* 2009; **40**: 179–91.

Lee MC, Eberson CP. Growth and development of the child's hip. *Orthop Clin N Am* 2006; **37**: 119–32.

Resnick D. *Diagnosis of bone and joint disorders*, 4th ed. Philadelphia: WB Saunders; 2002.

Slovis TL. *Caffey's pediatric diagnostic imaging*, 11th ed. Philadelphia: Mosby Elsevier; 2008: 2853–8.

Waite BL, Krabak BJ. Examination and treatment of pediatric injuries of the hip and pelvis. *Phys Med Rehabil Clin N Am* 2008; **19**: 305–18.

Packet 4 Case 4 Question

KIAT TAN

Clinical history

A 66-year-old female with a history of congenital hydrocephalus treated by ventriculo-atrial shunting presents with sudden onset shortness of breath.

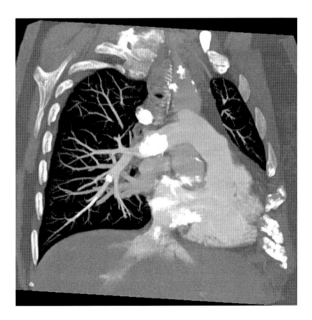

Figure 4.4.1

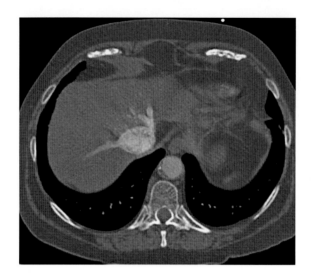

Figure 4.4.2

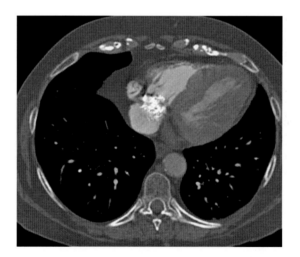

Figure 4.4.3

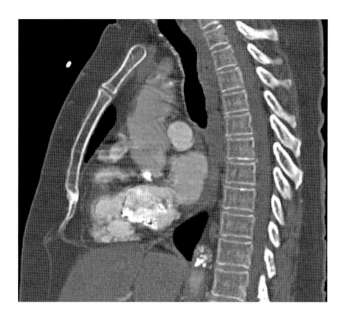

Figure 4.4.4

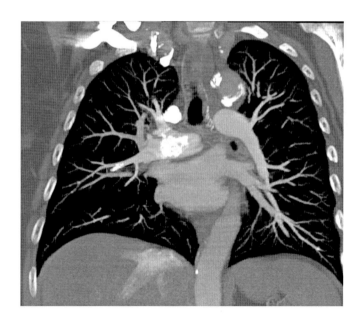

Figure 4.4.5

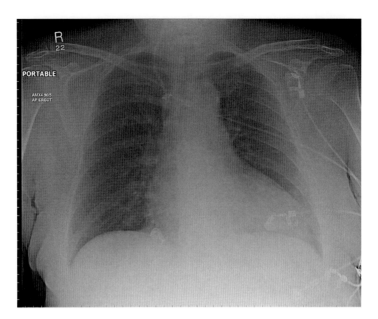

Figure 4.4.6

Answers to follow on page 140

Packet 4 Case 4 Answer

Model answer

Examination
- Computed tomography pulmonary angiogram (CTPA).
- Chest radiograph (portable).

Findings and interpretation

Chest radiograph
- The chest is clear.
- No pneumothorax.
- Ventriculo-atrial shunt present in situ.

CTPA
- Ventriculo-atrial shunt in situ (Figure 4.4.6).
- The inferior vena cava is dilated with reflux of contrast into the hepatic veins, consistent with raised right heart pressure (Figure 4.4.2).
- Large calcified embolus in the right main pulmonary artery, with a smaller more distal embolus (Figure 4.4.5).
- Calcification of the right atrium/tricuspid valve area (Figure 4.4.3).

Diagnosis
Multiple calcified pulmonary emboli originating from the right atrium/tricuspid valve area and resulting in raised right heart pressure, related to the previous ventriculo-atrial shunt. There are no real differential diagnoses for this appearance.

Management
- Needs echocardiogram to quantify cardiac function and right-sided cardiac pressures.
- The case needs to be discussed with the cardiologists and neurosurgeons.

In this case
This case illustrates the importance of viewing CTPA with a wide window (Figure 4.4.7). The embolus cannot be visualized on the normal soft tissue window (Figure 4.4.8).

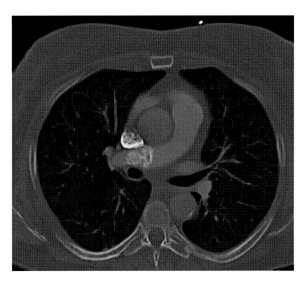

Figure 4.4.7 CT with IV contrast viewed on wide windows.

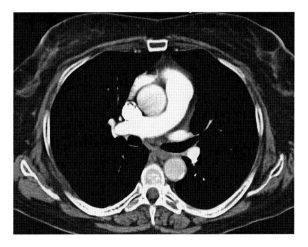

Figure 4.4.8 CT with IV contrast. The calcified thrombus is not visible.

The supervising radiologist also arranged for the patient to have a delayed CT of the chest to confirm the calcific nature of the embolus (Figure 4.4.9).

The patient had a subsequent echocardiogram which confirmed the presence of calcification in the right atrium near the tip of the V-A shunt. It was decided to adopt a conservative approach in the treatment of this patient and the V-A shunt was left in situ.

Ventriculo-atrial shunting

CSF shunting was a procedure that revolutionized the treatment of hydrocephalus. CSF shunting involves the formation of an accessory pathway for CSF flow in order to bypass the natural drainage system, which has become obstructed. The obstruction can be communicating or non-communicating. There are three types of CSF shunt procedures that are performed: ventriculo-peritoneal (V-P), ventriculo-atrial (V-A) and lumbo-peritoneal (L-P). Commonly V-P and V-A shunts are performed and in

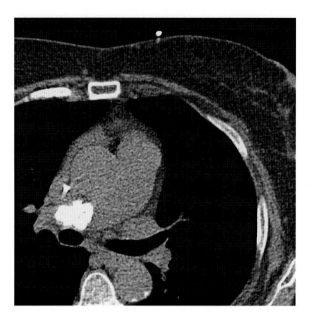

Figure 4.4.9 Delayed CT demonstrating calcified thrombus in the right main pulmonary artery.

the case of ventriculo-atrial shunting, the CSF is shunted into the right atrium of the heart via the shunt line, where the CSF is directly absorbed by the circulation. L-P shunting involves CSF shunting from the lumbar subarachnoid space into the peritoneal cavity, the main advantage being complete extracranial surgical management with minimization of intracranial complications.

The V-A shunts have a pressure-regulated valve placed under the scalp. The valve is connected to siliconized radio-opaque rubber catheters of very low tissue reactivity. These in turn connect the valve to one of the lateral ventricles superiorly, and inferiorly to the right atrium. The inferior shunt line is commonly introduced into either the right common facial vein or the right internal jugular vein leading into the superior vena cava and into the right atrium. A post-operative chest examination is taken as a baseline for future comparative studies. When V-A shunts become non-functional a radiographic survey of the entire length of the valve and tubing should be performed to assess for lucencies, kinks or separations.

V-A shunts are associated with atrial thrombosis and chronic pulmonary thromboembolism, which can result in secondary pulmonary hypertension. The catheter is a foreign body which promotes the formation of thrombus in situ, at its entry point either in the jugular vein or within the right atrium. This can lead to pulmonary embolism and, if chronic, can lead to secondary pulmonary hypertension. There is a high mortality rate of 50–100% in patients who develop secondary pulmonary hypertension complicating V-A shunts.

Shunt nephritis, an immune-mediated disease, is another rare and late complication resulting from chronic infection of the V-A shunt by organisms such as *Staphylococcus epidermidis*. Chronic low-grade bacteraemia is an indication for removal of the shunt line. Other potential complications of shunts include: subdural collections/haemorrhage due to rapid collapse of the ventricles leading to rupture of bridging meningeal veins, upward displacement of the brainstem and cerebellum secondary to decompression, and acute pulmonary oedema secondary to rapid fluid shift.

Owing to the reasons outlined above, the procedure has been superseded by ventriculo-peritoneal drainage.

References

Favara BE, Paul PN. Thromboembolism and cor pulmonale complicating ventriculoatrial shunts. *JAMA* 1967; **199**: 671–88.

Haasnoot K, van Vught AJ. Pulmonary hypertension complicating a ventriculoatrial shunt. *Eur J Pediatr* 2005; **151**: 748–50.

Kurlander GJ, Chua GT. Roentgenology of ventriculo-atrial shunts for the treatment of hydrocephalus. *AJR* 1967; **101**(1): 157–67.

Vernet O, Rilliet B. Late complications of ventriculoatrial or ventriculoperitoneal shunts. *The Lancet* 2001; **358**(9293): 1569–70.

Packet 4 Case 5 Question

MANDY WILLIAMS

Clinical history

A 32-year-old woman with haemolytic uraemic syndrome and hypertension presents with a seizure and visual disturbance.

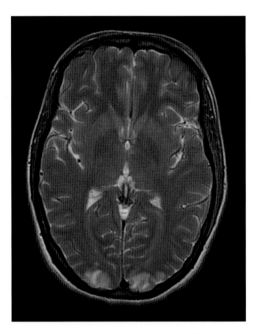

Figure 4.5.1 Pre-treatment MRI.

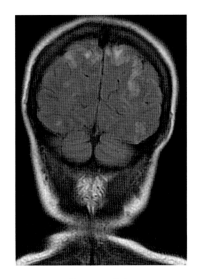

Figure 4.5.2

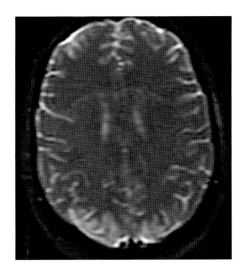

Figure 4.5.3

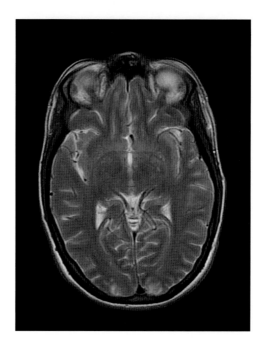

Figure 4.5.4 Post-treatment MRI.

Answers to follow on page 148

Packet 4 Case 5 Answer

Model answer

Examination
MRI brain: non-contrast:

- Axial T2-weighted (Figure 4.5.1).
- Coronal FLAIR (fluid attenuated inversion recovery) sequences (Figure 4.5.2).
- Diffusion weighted image (DWI) (Figure 4.5.3).
- Axial T2-weighted (Figure 4.5.4).

Observations and interpretations
- There is high signal in both occipital lobes and parietal lobes. This is seen most clearly on the FLAIR imaging and is centred on the subcortical white matter.
- There is sulcal effacement and mild mass effect associated with these changes, which are bilateral and asymmetrical.
- The CSF spaces are normal.
- There is no midline shift, no extra axial collections.
- The remainder of the brain appears normal.

Interpretation
The high signal represents oedema within the tissues. No associated mass or infiltration is seen. This is therefore likely to be a benign process rather than a malignant one.

Diagnosis
Posterior reversible encephalopathy syndrome (PRES).

Differential diagnosis
- Cerebritis.
- Stroke.

Management
Early diagnosis is important as the condition, if treated early, is completely reversible; however, delay can lead to infarction.

Subtle early changes are visible on CT scan with low density seen in the occipital and parietal lobes with associated sulcal effacement. This is seen in the white matter only, differentiating this condition from infarction, which involves the grey and white matter.

In this case the patient's hypertension was aggressively managed and a follow-up MRI 1 week later revealed almost complete resolution of the changes.

Posterior reversible encephalopathy syndrome

This is a clinicoradiological entity characterized by visual disturbance, headaches, altered mental status and seizures. Patients have an acute or subacute presentation and similar imaging findings regardless of the underlying cause. The main common denominator in cases is severe hypertension. In some patients the blood pressure is mildly elevated or normal at initial presentation. The exact mechanism is not clear, and the hypothesis is a reduced blood–brain barrier with increased permeability of fluid leading to vasogenic oedema.

The clue to the diagnosis is the presence of cortical and subcortical white matter oedema in patients with severe hypertension. Patchy enhancement with gadolinium is observed on T1-weighted imaging.

Common causes of PRES
- Hypertension.
- Pre-eclampsia.
- Drugs – chemotherapy agents and immunosuppressants: cyclosporin A, bevacizumab (Avastin) a recombinant humanized monoclonal IgG1 antibody for treatment of renal cell carcinoma.
- Severe hypercalcaemia.
- Autoimmune diseases: systemic lupus erythematosus, haemolytic uraemic syndrome.
- Severe sepsis.
- Renal disease.

By aggressive prompt treatment of the cause the condition is fully reversible without any residual atrophy or gliotic change. Usually no anticonvulsants are required long term.

The neuroimaging findings are of reversible vasogenic oedema without infarction.

MRI reveals white matter oedema in the occipital lobes and parietal lobes and occasionally more anterior structures are affected. Haemorrhage is not a typical feature and this helps to differentiate PRES from a primary infarction with haemorrhagic transformation or venous infarction.

Imaging features
- Patchy symmetrical bilateral subcortical vasogenic oedema.
- Posterior regions are predominantly affected.
- Complete clinical and radiographic resolution.

CT
- Low attenuation in the occipital lobes, involving the white matter.
- No enhancement post contrast unless infarction has occurred.

MRI

Typical imaging features
- Subcortical white matter vasogenic oedema best demonstrated on the T2-weighted sequences and high signal on FLAIR. FLAIR increases the conspicuity of lesions.

- Gyriform high signal.
- DWI slight increase or isointense signal.
- Increased (bright) diffusion coefficient (ADC) apparent.
- No enhancement or patchy enhancement on T1-weighted sequence with contrast.
- Earliest resolution of changes has been reported in 5 days and as late as weeks to years later. Average range is several days to weeks for resolution of changes.

Atypical imaging features

- Anterior involvement: frontal lobes.
- Cortical lesions: grey matter involvement.
- Haemorrhage: subarachnoid, intraparenchymal or into lesions.
- Contrast enhancement.
- Other areas can be involved: basal ganglia, thalami, cerebellum, brainstem. In such atypical cases without parietoccipital involvement, other causes need to be excluded, e.g. central pontine myelinosis or encephalomyelitis.
- Unilaterality.
- Recurrent episodes can occur in the same patient.

References

Casey SO, Sampaio RC, Michel E, Truwit CL. Posterior reversible encephalopathy syndrome: utility of fluid attenuated inversion recovery MR imaging in the detection of cortical and subcortical lesions. *AJNR* 2000; **21**: 1199–206.

Glusker P, Recht L, Lane B. Reversible posterior leukoencephalopathy syndrome and bevacizumab. *N Engl J Med* 2006; **354**(9): 980–2.

Lee VH, Wijidicks EFM, Manno EM, Rabinstein AA. Clinical spectrum of reversible posterior leukoencephalopathy syndrome. *Arch Neurol* 2008; **65**(2): 205–10.

McKinney MA, Short J, Truwit CL et al. Posterior reversible encephalopathy syndrome: incidence of atypical regions of involvement and imaging findings. *AJR* 2007; **189**: 904–12.

Port J, Beauchamp N. Reversible intracerebral pathological entities mediated by vascular autoregulatory dysfunction. *RadioGraphics* 1998; **18**: 353–67.

Schwartz RB, Feske SK, Polak JF et al. Preeclampsia–eclampsia: clinical and neuroradiographic correlates and insights into the pathogenesis of hypertensive encephalopathy. *Radiology* 2000; **217**: 371–6.

Packet 4 Case 6 Question

NEIL COLLIN

Clinical history

A diabetic female presents with abdominal pain and low-grade pyrexia.

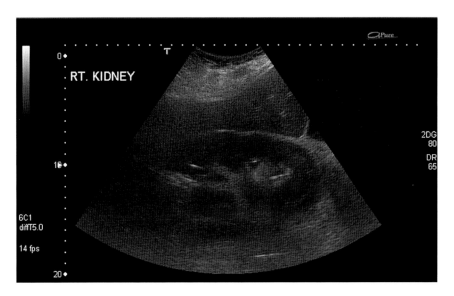

Figure 4.6.1

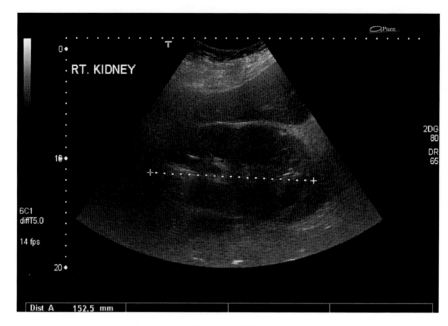

Figure 4.6.2

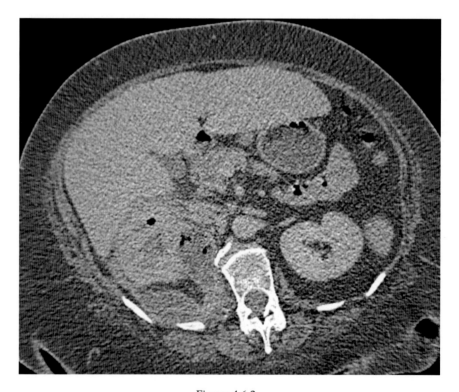

Figure 4.6.3

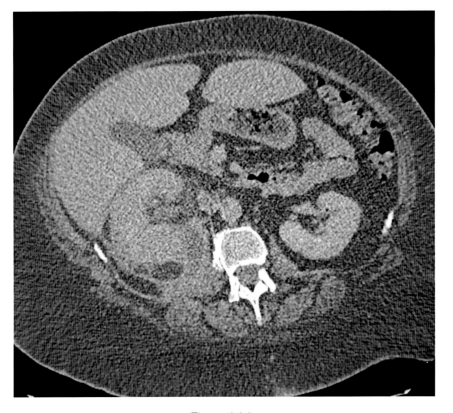

Figure 4.6.4

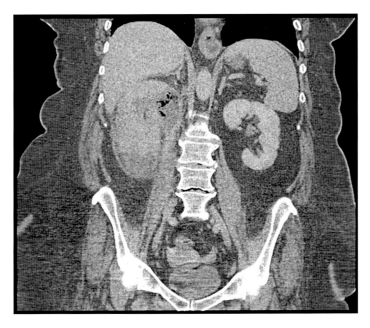

Figure 4.6.5

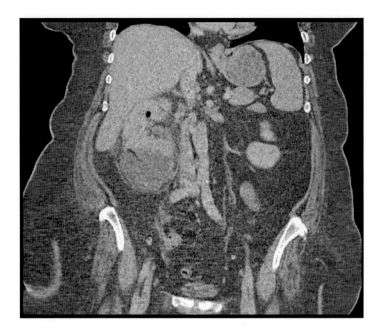

Figure 4.6.6

Answers to follow on page 156

Packet 4 Case 6 Answer

Model answer

Findings and interpretations

Renal ultrasound (Figures 4.6.1 and 4.6.2)
- Right kidney is enlarged (15 cm).
- Low echogenicity, loss of cortico-medullary differentiation.
- Several small echogenic foci in renal parenchyma, with no acoustic shadows.

Contrast-enhanced CT abdomen axial and coronal sections (Figures 4.6.3 to 4.6.6)
- Right kidney demonstrates an enlarged low density area in the lower pole.
- Multiple gas locules and fluid collections within renal parenchyma.
- Perinephric fluid and gas.
- No hydronephrosis.
- No renal calculi.
- Liver, spleen and left kidney grossly normal.

Diagnosis
- Emphysematous pyelonephritis.
- Renal and perinephric abscess.

Management
- Admit, antibiotics, tight control of diabetes.
- Percutaneous drainage of the focal collections at the lower pole of the right kidney and in the perinephric space may be necessary.
- Non-response to medical management may necessitate surgical drainage or nephrectomy.

In this case
The patient made a good initial recovery with optimization of diabetic control and IV antibiotics. At 1 week residual low-grade fever prompted a repeat CT that showed a small residual collection at the lower pole of the kidney. This was drained percutaneously under CT guidance with a good result.

Emphysematous pyelonephritis

Urinary tract infections are very common and only rarely do they lead to emphysematous pyelonephritis (EPN). EPN is a life-threatening condition and is usually associated with poorly controlled diabetes. Less common associations include any cause of immunosuppression, polycystic kidney disease and end stage renal failure. It can occur in non-diabetic patients with urinary tract obstruction from stones, tumour or sloughed papillae. Transplanted kidneys are more susceptible to emphysematous pyelonephritis because of associated risk factors such as diabetes and immunosuppression.

Escherichia coli is the causative organism in most patients with *Klebsiella* species being the second commonest organism. *Proteus, pseudomonas* and *Streptococcus* species have also been reported, and mixed organisms occur in 10%.

The clinical presentation is similar to acute pyelonephritis; however it often follows a more severe clinical course and mortality is high if left untreated.

Severe necrotizing infection results in gas formation within the collecting system, renal parenchyma and/or perinephric tissues.

Several staging systems have been proposed including the following by Huang et al:

- Class 1 – gas confined to the collecting system.
- Class 2 – gas confined to the renal parenchyma alone.
- Class 3A – perinephric extension of gas or abscess.
- Class 3B – extension of gas beyond Gerota's fascia.
- Class 4 – bilateral EPN or EPN in solitary kidney.

Prompt antibiotic treatment and optimization of diabetic control are essential. In less severe cases (class 1 and 2) antibiotics and percutaneous drainage of focal collections and insertion of nephrostomy to decompress an obstructed system are usually sufficient. Class 3 and 4 may respond to conservative management but are more likely to require surgical drainage or nephrectomy. Early surgical and ICU review is recommended as diabetic ketoacidosis (DKA) often results and failure to respond to medical management may require nephrectomy.

Imaging features

Plain films
- Gas within the renal beds or overlying the renal fossa. Gas in a crescentic shape may be seen within Gerota's fascia. This is an ominous sign, indicating a more severe stage and suggests renal necrosis.
- Radio-opaque renal stones may be seen, but this is a non-specific finding. It is seen in a spectrum of causes of pyelonephritis (see case example below).
- Obscuration of the ipsilateral psoas shadow.

Ultrasound
- Obstruction may occur and is denoted by hydronephrosis.
- Enlarged kidneys.
- Echogenic foci, different to stones, indicating gas. The distal shadowing shows reverberations and low-level echoes.

CT
- Imaging modality of choice.
- Enlarged kidneys.
- Linear streaks or bubbles of gas.
- Fluid collections.
- Gas-fluid levels.

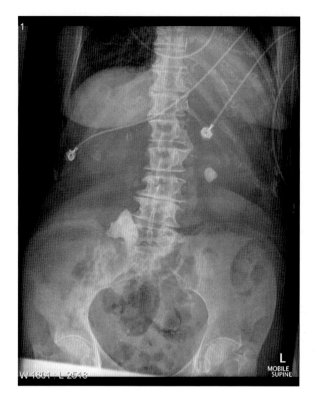

Figure 4.6.7

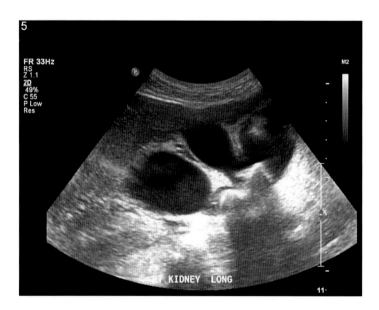

Figure 4.6.8

- Focal tissue necrosis.
- Abscess formation.

Nuclear medicine
- Used to assess and quantify renal function.

A further case example of obstructive pyelonephritis

Figures 4.6.7 and 4.6.8 are images of another patient who was admitted to ICU with urinary sepsis. This was due to obstruction from bilateral large renal calculi obstructing the renal pelvis.

This is an abdominal plain radiograph showing a large right stag horn calculus and a smaller one on the left. There was no improvement in the clinical course despite full medical management on ICU. Further imaging with an ultrasound examination demonstrated severe hydronephrosis secondary to a large calculus in the renal pelvis.

References

Craig WD, Wagner BJ, Travis M. From the archives of the AFIP: Pyelonephritis: radiologic-pathologic review. *RadioGraphics* 2008; **28**: 255–76.

Grayson DE, Abbott RM, Levy AD, Sherman PM. Emphysematous infections of the abdomen and pelvis: a pictorial review. *RadioGraphics* 2002; **22**: 543–61.

Huang JJ, Tseng CC. Emphysematous pyelonephritis: clinicoradiological classification, management, prognosis, and pathogenesis. *Arch Intern Med* 2000; **160**(6): 797–805.

Nawaz Kan A. *Emphysematous pyelonephritis*. Jan 2008. Available at: http://www.emedicine.com/radio/TOPIC244.HTM

Packet 5 Case 1 Question

KATE TAYLOR-ROBINSON

Clinical history

Painful swollen leg for 1 month.

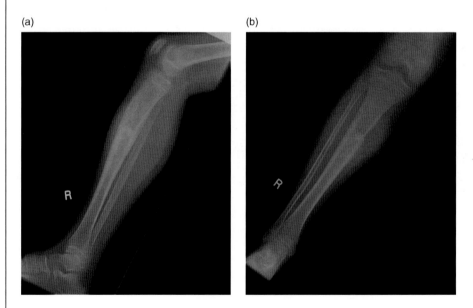

Figure 5.1.1

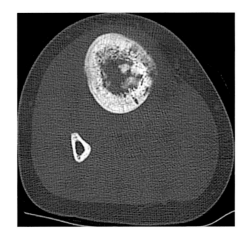

Figure 5.1.2

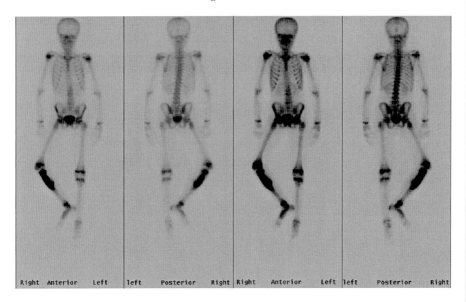

Figure 5.1.3

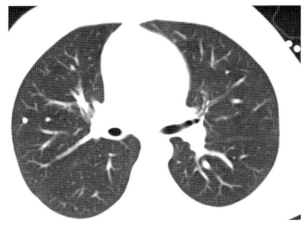

Figure 5.1.4

(a)

(b)

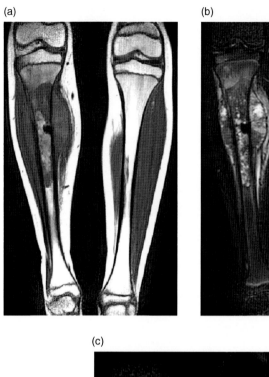

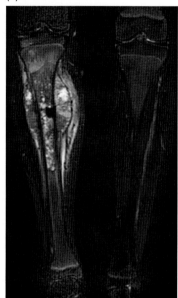

(c)

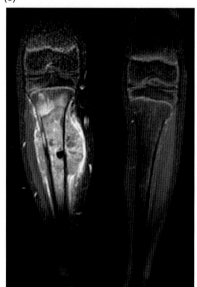

Figure 5.1.5

Answers to follow on page 164

Packet 5 Case 1 Answer

Model answer

Examinations
- Plain radiographs of the tibia and fibula (Figure 5.1.1).
- Axial CT image of right tibia and fibula (Figure 5.1.2).
- 99mTc MDP bone scan (Figure 5.1.3).

Observations and interpretations

CT thorax–lung windows (Figure 5.1.4)
- Plain radiographs and CT demonstrate a mixed sclerotic and lucent lesion of the proximal right tibia.
- There is a permeative pattern of bone destruction. There is an elevated and interrupted periosteal reaction with a Codman's triangle demonstrating rapid growth. The zone of transition is indistinct. There is associated soft tissue swelling.
- The bone scan confirms that the lesion is solitary within the skeleton and shows marked osteoblastic activity.
- The lung CT demonstrates a few small parenchymal nodules most likely consistent with metastases within this clinical context.

Diagnosis
Osteosarcoma of the right tibia with lung metastases.

Differential diagnosis
- Ewing's sarcoma.
- Osteomyelitis.
- Other causes of pulmonary nodules, e.g. granulomas due to previous TB.

Management
- An MRI of the affected bone including the joint above and below the lesion is indicated to define local extent of the disease and pre-surgical assessment/planning.

- Biopsy should only be undertaken with the guidance of the regional referral centre for sarcoma taking into account the surgical approach. Alternatively biopsy may be performed by the regional sarcoma centre.
- A review of the CT thorax using mediastinal and bone windows should be undertaken to ascertain whether the nodules are calcified.

Osteosarcoma

Osteosarcoma is one of two most common malignant bone tumours in children and teenagers. Osteosarcoma is most common between 10 and 15 years of age, with a male predilection. In the younger population, they tend to arise de novo and commonly occur within the metaphyses of long bones, the bones around the knee joint and the proximal humerus.

A second peak occurs in the older population, usually those older than 40 years. In this age group, they tend to arise in areas of prior radiation exposure or malignant transformation of Paget's disease (1% of patients with Paget's). The axial skeleton is a common location compared to metaphyses in the younger population.

Pain is a common presenting symptom, with or without swelling. Sometimes there may be a history of trauma, which can be a distracting feature in the history. However repeat presentation with persistent pain despite rest and analgesia are worrying clinical features as well as night pain.

Osteosarcomas are a heterogeneous group of soft tissue tumours, and the under-lying genetic aetiology in de novo osteosarcomas is not currently understood. No consistent genetic alteration has been identified and it appears random according to the current understanding. Some of the genetic alterations that have been found include p53, and the MDM2 genes.

The plain radiograph is an excellent first-line imaging investigation.
Features to look for include:

- Destructive lesion.
- Malignant periosteal reaction:
  - Sun-burst appearance – spiculated and disrupted, like sun rays
  - Codman's triangle – this is caused by elevation of the periosteum from the underlying bone.
  - Onion skin appearance – lamellated.
- Soft tissue mass.

Then further assessment with cross-sectional imaging is required.

MR is the next line of investigation in characterizing soft tissue tumours further. It will assess joint, soft tissue, intramedullary involvement and the extension of the tumour. It is desirable to perform the MR prior to biopsy, as post-interventional changes will make reviewing the imaging more challenging.

Usually tumour is seen as:

- Low signal on T1-weighted sequence
- Low signal on T2-weighted sequence
- High signal on STIR sequence
- Enhancement of tumour on post contrast.

Investigation with chest CT assessing for lung metastases is appropriate. Pulmonary metastases are the most common presentation of distant spread. They occur in 15% of all cases and in 2% at presentation and often calcify. In approximately 20% of cases of lung metastases there is uptake of MDP on bone scans. Lung metastases tend to be subpleural and may cavitate, causing pneumothorax.

Current treatment is surgery with a wide clear surgical margin and pre- and post-operative chemotherapy.

Prognostic markers are

- The response to chemotherapy; this is the strongest predictor for survival.
- The presence of pulmonary metastases or recurrent disease.
- Size and location of the tumour.

The response to chemotherapy is graded by the percentage of tumour necrosis on histology. A response of greater than 90% tumour necrosis can equate to 80–90% long-term survival and a dramatic decrease in survival rate to less than 15% for response of less than 90% tumour necrosis. In this heterogeneous group of tumours, some lesions will be chemoresistant and one of the goals of current research is to predict who would be poor responders.

Post treatment, the soft tissue component of an osteosarcoma usually ossifies.

If there is local availability, FDG–PET is highly sensitive in the detection of local recurrence in the post therapy setting.

MRI (Figures 5.1.5a–c) demonstrates the local extent of the soft tissue and bone mass in the right proximal tibia with mixed cystic and sclerotic components and extensive enhancement post gadolinium.

References

Hayden JB, Hoang BH. Osteosarcoma: basic science and clinical implications. *Orthop Clin N Am* 2006; **37**: 1–7.

Hwang S, Panicek DM. The evolution of musculoskeletal tumor imaging. *Radiol Clin N Am* 2009; **47**: 435–53.

Lane F. *Diagnostic imaging: pediatrics*, 1st ed. Amirsys Inc. Donnelly/Elsevier; 2005: 78–81.

Nazemi KJ, Malempati S. Emergency department presentation of childhood cancer. *Emerg Med Clin N Am* 2009; **27**: 477–95.

Wootton-Gorges S. MR imaging of primary bone tumors and tumor-like conditions in children. *Magn Reson Imaging Clin N Am* 2009; **17**: 469–87.

Wu JMW, Montgomery E. Classification and pathology. *Surgical Clin of N Am* 2008; **88**: 483–520.

Packet 5 Case 2 Question

JOANNA KASZNIA-BROWN

Clinical history

Increasing headaches with tinnitus and right-sided hearing loss. Paraesthesia experienced in the right facial area, left arm and both lower limbs.

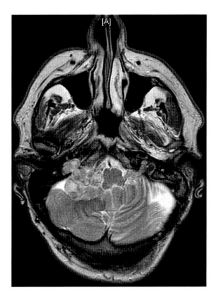

Figure 5.2.1

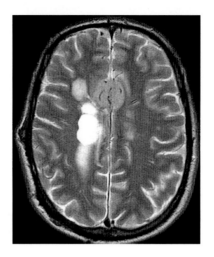

Figure 5.2.2

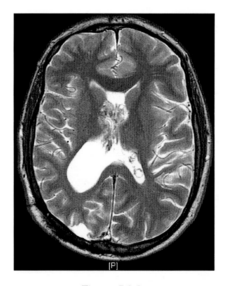

Figure 5.2.3

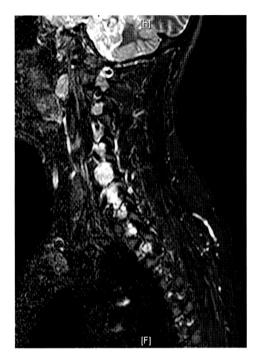

Figure 5.2.4

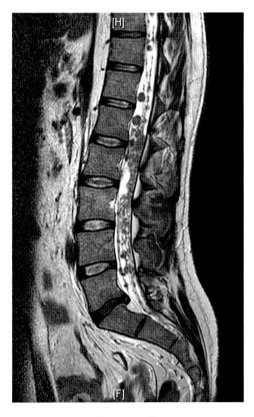

Figure 5.2.5

Packet 5 Case 2 Answer

Model answer

Examination
- MRI brain – axial T2-weighted images (Figures 5.2.1, 5.2.2 and 5.2.3).
- MRI cervical spine – sagittal STIR images (Figure 5.2.4).
- MRI lumbar spine – sagittal T2-weighted image (Figure 5.2.5).

Findings

MRI brain
- Bilateral lobulated soft tissue masses in the cerebello-pontine angles. They appear isointense on the T2-weighted sequence and extend along the vestibulocochlear nerves into the enlarged internal acoustic canals.
- Lesion in the right CPA measures 5 × 4.5 cm and causes a marked distortion of the right middle cerebellar peduncle and mass effect on the right cerebellar hemisphere.
- Well-defined interhemispheric soft tissue mass in the region of frontal horns of the lateral ventricles. It appears homogeneous and hyperintense to the brain parenchyma on T2-weighted imaging. There is mild oedema in the surrounding white matter (more advanced on the right).
- Multiple irregular lesions in the lateral ventricles. The biggest lesion is isointense on T2-weighted sequence.
- Dilatation of the posterior horn and posterior body of the right lateral ventricle.

MRI cervical spine
- Multiple well-defined lesions in the upper and mid levels of the cervical spine, closely related to the nerve roots. They appear hyperintense on the STIR sequence.
- Enlargement of multiple neural foramina of the cervical spine.

MRI lumbar spine
- Multiple small round well-defined lesions (isointense on T2-weighted sequence) arising from the nerve roots along the cauda equina.
- Multiple well-defined lesions (isointense on T2-weighted sequence) arising in the conus medullaris and causing it to expand.

Interpretations

Multiple intracranial and spinal lesions:

- Bilateral vestibular (acoustic) schwannomas
- Intraventricular and interhemispheric meningiomas
- Spinal neurofibromas/schwannomas
- Ependymomas in the conus.

Diagnosis

Neurofibromatosis type 2 (central).

Differential diagnosis

No differential diagnosis for this condition.

Management

- Referral to neurology team.
- Family surveillance ± screening.

Neurofibromatosis

Neurofibromatosis 2 (NF2) is a rare autosomal dominant syndrome, associated with a mutation of the NF2 gene, located on the long arm of chromosome 22 (22q12 abnormality). The estimated incidence of NF2 is 1:37 000 per year and about half of cases are a result of new mutations.

Neurofibromatosis 2 is characterized by multiple schwannomas, meningiomas and ependymomas.

The most common tumour associated with the syndrome is the vestibulocochlear schwannoma. Ten to twenty-five percent of patients presenting with this tumour will be found to have NF2.

Bilateral acoustic schwannomas allow a presumptive diagnosis of type 2 neurofibromatosis.

Typically, the diagnosis of NF2 is made in the 2nd and 3rd decade of life, with a peak incidence in the 20s. Approximately 45% of patients present with symptoms of eight and seventh nerve schwannomas such as hearing loss, tinnitus, balance impairment and weakness of the muscles supplied by the facial nerve.

In the paediatric population, ocular abnormalities are the most common clinical presentation, whilst other lesions are discovered by family screening.

Part of the family screening will involve a contrast-enhanced MRI of the brain and entire spine. Contrast examination is important for detecting small schwannomas, particularly spinal nerve roots and small intraparenchymal ependymomas.

Diagnostic criteria for NF2

1. Bilateral vestibular schwannomas.
2. First-degree relative with NF2 and one vestibular schwannoma or two of the following: meningioma, schwannoma, glioma, neurofibroma, posterior lens opacity or cerebral calcification.
3. Two of the following – unilateral vestibular schwannoma, multiple meningiomas, either schwannoma, glioma, neurofibroma, posterior lens opacity or cerebral calcification.

Eighty-five percent of acoustic schwannomas arise from the vestibular portion of the eighth nerve and 15% from the cochlear portion. Acoustic schwannoma is a round mass extending along the internal acoustic canal (IAC) and forms an acute angle with the dural surface of the petrous bone (a meningioma forms an obtuse angle with the dura giving rise to the so-called 'dural tail'). Schwannomas extend into the IAC, causing its enlargement in 70–90% of cases. Degenerative changes (cysts and haemorrhage) are common with tumours bigger than 2–3 cm.

Schwannomas are usually isodense with brain parenchyma on an unenhanced CT scan with uniform dense enhancement with intravenous contrast. Asymmetry or enlargement of the IACs can be suggestive but not sensitive.

Large tumours can be slightly hypodense with peripheral, ring enhancement secondary to central necrosis. They normally do not contain calcification. A neuroma is typically iso- or slightly hypointense on T1-weighted imaging and similar to CT, shows strong enhancement with post IV contrast (two-thirds solid, a third ring or heterogeneous). Ninety percent of neuromas are hyperintense on T2-weighted sequence. The differential diagnosis of acoustic neuroma includes: meningioma, other schwannomas – fifth or seventh cranial nerves, epidermoid or arachnoid cyst and metastasis.

References

Aoki S, Barkovich AJ, Nishimura K et al. Neurofibromatosis types 1 and 2: cranial MR findings. *Radiology* 1989; **172**(2): 527–34.

Gutmann DH, Aylsworth A, Carey JC et al. The diagnostic evaluation and multidisciplinary management of neurofibromatosis 1 and neurofibromatosis 2. *JAMA* 1997; **278**(1): 51–7.

Patronas NJ, Courcoutsakis N, Bromley CM et al. Intramedullary and spinal canal tumours in patients with neurofibromatosis 2: MR imaging findings and correlation with genotype. *Radiology* 2001; **218**: 434–42.

Packet 5 Case 3 Question

MARC WILLIAMS

Clinical history

A 55-year-old male presents with headaches and right-sided weakness.

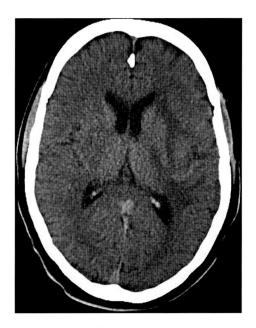

Figure 5.3.1

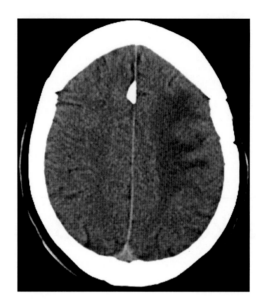

Figure 5.3.2

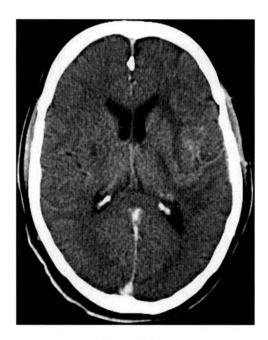

Figure 5.3.3

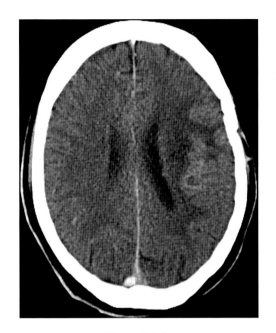

Figure 5.3.4

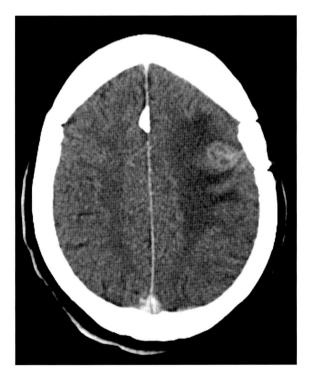

Figure 5.3.5

Packet 5 Case 3 Answer

Model answer

Observations and interpretations

The figures are five selected axial images from a CT head examination. Figures 5.3.1 and 5.3.2 are pre-contrast and Figures 5.3.3, 5.3.4 and 5.3.5 are post-contrast. There is a mass in the left frontal lobe, in the region of the external capsule, with surrounding oedema. There is a second lesion towards the vertex, again in the left frontal lobe, which also demonstrates surrounding oedema. Both masses demonstrate contrast enhancement. The midline appears central.

Principal diagnosis and differential diagnosis

The most likely diagnosis in a patient with multiple, intracranial masses would be cerebral metastases. This diagnosis would be strengthened in a patient with a known primary tumour. The differential diagnosis is limited but would include multicentric glioblastoma multiforme and lymphoma.

Management

The report should be urgently communicated to the clinician and an urgent neuro-surgical referral undertaken. An MRI scan of the brain will be needed. Since there is likely to be concern that the appearances could be due to metastatic disease, a CT scan of the chest, abdomen and pelvis may be requested prior to a biopsy. Dexamethasone can be given to reduce the vasogenic oedema.

The diagnosis in this case is multicentric glioblastoma multiforme, which was confirmed by biopsy.

Glioblastoma multiforme

Glioblastoma multiforme (GBM) is the most common glial cell and primary cerebral tumour with an incidence of approximately 2–3 new cases per 100 000 people per year. The aetiology remains unclear though numerous genetic abnormalities have been demonstrated.

GBM primarily affects adults with a peak incidence of 45–70 years and most often arises de novo, i.e. not from the degeneration of a lower grade astrocytoma, which tends to occur in younger patients. GBMs are most often located in the subcortical white matter of the cerebral hemispheres, the most common location being the fronto-temporal region. The occipital lobes are usually spared.

GBM is one of the most malignant of all neoplasms and the most malignant of the glioma group. GBM often demonstrates marked microvascular proliferation, infiltration and necrosis. Tumours are often ill-defined and have a tendency to invade locally along white matter pathways, such as the corpus callosum, giving rise to the so-called 'butterfly glioma'. Such spread may also cause multicentric GBMs, which occurs in 2–5% of cases. Spread to the CSF and extracerebral metastases occur rarely.

Despite an often-short history of symptoms, tumours are usually large at diagnosis. The prognosis is therefore uniformly poor and the treatment palliative, which includes surgery, radiotherapy and chemotherapy. Even with maximal treatment, tumours typically recur and the median survival is approximately 12 months. In some patients, where the tumour is located in a vital region of the brain and when the tumour has no defined margin, or the patient is unfit for maximal therapy, stereotactic biopsy followed by radiation therapy may be considered. In such circumstances, median survival is estimated to be in the region of 27–47 weeks.

Patients present most commonly with a progressive neurological deficit, headache, which is often worse in the morning and associated with nausea and vomiting. New onset seizures and changes in personality and concentration are other commonly presenting signs.

Differential diagnoses to consider include:

- Cerebral metastasis – may be solitary or multiple
- Cerebral abscess (ring enhancement thinner than GBM)
- Primary CNS lymphoma (periventricular in location; it can be difficult and may require biopsy, MR spectroscopy or PET to aid in the diagnosis)
- 'Tumefactive' demyelination (usually seen as an incomplete ring enhancement).

On CT scans, GBM is typically an irregular, poorly defined, iso- or hypodense lesion, which can demonstrate homogeneous, heterogeneous or ring-like enhancement. There is central hypodensity representing central necrosis. There is usually associated cerebral oedema and there may be considerable mass effect. The other consideration for the appearance of the surrounding low density is that it may represent tumour infiltration. There can be tumour extension across the corpus callosum to involve the contralateral hemisphere.

On MRI, GBM is usually of low signal intensity on T1-weighted images and high signal intensity on T2-weighted images, with surrounding vasogenic oedema best visualized on T2-weighted and FLAIR sequences. The oedema extends along central white matter tracts. Tumour extension across the corpus callosum or other white matter tracts, anterior and posterior commissure, can be clearly demonstrated. Post-contrast T1-weighted images usually demonstrate tumour enhancement (thick and irregular margins), particularly related to the periphery of the tumour, and separate tumour nodules may also be apparent. Following surgery, MRI is undertaken to determine the extent of surgical resection and as a base line scan. Contrast enhancement at this stage or future stages reflects residual or recurrent tumour.

It can be difficult to differentiate recurrent tumour from radiation necrosis following treatment. In order to help differentiate between these two diagnoses, positron emission tomography and magnetic resonance spectroscopy can be helpful. In recurrent GBM, magnetic resonance spectroscopy may demonstrate an increase in the choline creatine ratio, an increased lactate peak and decreased N-acetylaspartate peak. Despite this, functional imaging is not 100% accurate and histology may still be required if there is doubt about the diagnosis.

References

Dahnert W. *Radiology review manual*. Philadelphia: Lippincott, Williams & Wilkins; 2003: 282–3.

Glioblastoma multiforme. 12 Apr 2007. Available at: http://www.emedicine.com/MED/topic2692.htm

Omunro AMO, Leite CC, Mokhatari K, Delattre J-Y. Pitfalls in the diagnosis of brain tumours. *Lancet Neurol* 2006; **5**; 937–48.

Osborn A, Blaser S, Salzman K et al. *Diagnostic imaging: brain*. Amirsys/Elsevier; 2004. P I:6:20.

Packet 5 Case 4 Question

KIAT TAN

Clinical history

An elderly patient with lymphoma is undergoing chemotherapy. Response to treatment?

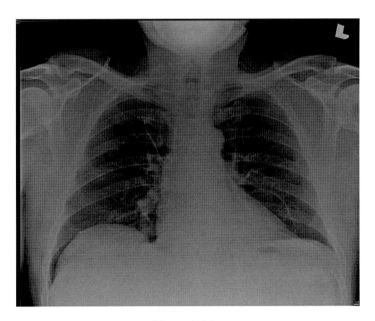

Figure 5.4.1

Packet 5 Case 4 Answer

Model answer

Examination
Chest radiograph.

Findings and interpretations
- There is a linear structure extending from the right upper lobe pulmonary artery to the left lower lobe artery.
- No Hickman or peripheral inserted central catheter (PICC) line is evident.
- Lungs are clear.
- Cardiac and mediastinal shadows are otherwise normal.

Diagnosis
PICC line embolus.

Differential diagnosis
Artefact on patient body surface.

Management
(1) Review old imaging.
(2) Lateral chest radiograph.
(3) Inform oncologists urgently.
(4) Arrange for the interventional radiologist to snare the line.

In this case
Comparison with old imaging is of the utmost importance. In this patient, the old film showed a left PICC line in situ (Figure 5.4.2). The oncology nurse practitioner was also rather alarmed to discover that the PICC line had disappeared from the left ante-cubital fossa! A lateral film, therefore, was not performed. The line was removed by the interventional radiologist on-call.

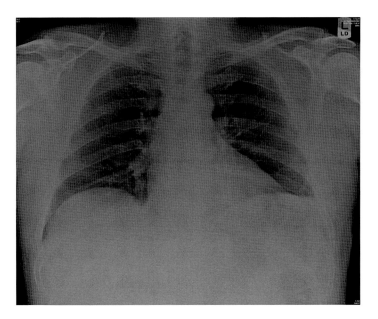

Figure 5.4.2

Line embolization

A peripheral inserted central catheter line is a long catheter inserted into a peripheral arm vein and tracked into the large veins just proximal to the right atrium. It is used when peripheral access is poor or when long-term delivery of drugs is necessary, e.g. long-term antibiotics for osteomyelitis treatment. It is used in both the paediatric and adult population. Complications related to PICC are: infections, tip migration, occlusion of the PICC, phlebitis, venous or right atrial perforation, catheter fracture and embolization.

Line embolization is a rare complication and there are usually no associated clinical symptoms. PICC line embolization can cause significant morbidity and mortality and prompt investigation should be initiated. Usually a chest radiograph can define the fracture site, but it is important to ensure the whole length of the catheter is seen. Fluoroscopy may then be required, if the catheter appears intact on the radiograph. Line exchange should be carried out in cases of suspected line damage.

Only a few studies have investigated the complications of PICC in adults and the paediatric population. In the study from the Hospital for Sick Children in Toronto, Canada an incidence of 6.7 in 1000 PICC lines were shown to have fractured or embolized.

In this study, embolization of the catheter fragment migrated to the pulmonary vascular system and they were retrieved successfully. The interventional radiologist can treat most cases of PICC line embolization without the need for open surgery. None of the patients had any long-term complications related to the PICC embolization.

PICC line embolization can be due to intrinsic catheter defects or human error. There is a current patient safety alert report for a specific PICC line (Arrow PICC line), which has been discovered to have intrinsic dysfunction. If the product's placement wire is damaged or cut during insertion, the outer coil can delaminate from the inner core, either breaking away or remaining in the catheter. It can subsequently migrate and lodge in the pulmonary artery. The fine coil of the wire is very difficult to visualize and can be missed on check radiographs.

References

Alert number 08_02, October 2008. *Peripherally inserted central catheter (PICC) device complications – guide wire retention.* Queensland Health, Queensland Government.

Chow LML, Lionel ML, Friedman JN et al. Peripherally inserted central catheter (PICC) fracture and embolization in the pediatric population. *J Pediatr* 2003; 141–4.

Monsuez JJ, Douard MC, Martin-Bouyer Y. Catheter fragments embolisation. *Angiology* 1997; **48**: 117–20.

Surov A, Buerke M, John E et al. Intravenous port embolisation: mechanisms, clinical features and management. *Angiology* 2008; **59**: 90–7.

Packet 5 Case 5 Question

NEIL COLLIN

Clinical history

A 20-year-old male presents with right flank pain.

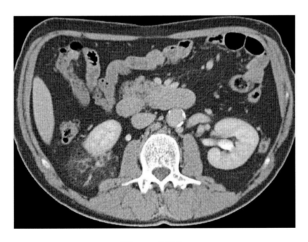

Figure 5.5.1

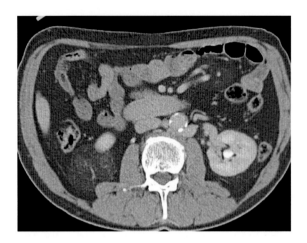

Figure 5.5.2

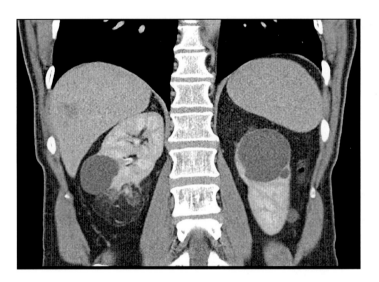

Figure 5.5.3

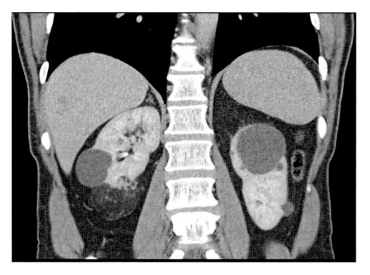

Figure 5.5.4

Packet 5 Case 5 Answer

Model answer

Examination
Contrast-enhanced CT abdomen, axial and coronal sections (Figures 5.5.1 to 5.5.4).

Findings and interpretations
Contrast-enhanced CT abdomen (venous phase):

- 5 cm lesion arising from the renal cortex of the lower pole of the right kidney
- Eccentric location, well-defined margins
- Predominantly fat density
- Serpiginous enhancing vessels within the mass
- No perinephric or retroperitoneal collection
- No adenopathy demonstrated
- Subtle low-density lesion right lobe of liver
- Simple cysts both kidneys.

Diagnosis
Right renal angiomyolipoma.
No evidence of acute bleed.

Differential diagnosis
Renal lipoma or fat-containing renal cell carcinoma (both rare).

Management
- Pre-emptive selective embolization or partial nephrectomy may be carried out to prevent risk of bleeding.
- History, examination: association with tuberous sclerosis.
- Usually benign, smaller lesions can be followed up with serial imaging. Ultrasound is preferable due to the radiation burden with CT imaging.

In this case

There were no other stigmata of tuberous sclerosis. The pain resolved and the urologists have planned serial ultrasound scans as follow-up for the patient.

Angiomyolipoma

Angiomyolipoma (AML) is a benign renal tumour made up, as the name suggests, of vascular, smooth muscle and fat components. The imaging finding of fat within a renal lesion is characteristic of AML, but not all AML will contain a macroscopic fat component. Other renal lesions that may contain fat are renal cell carcinomas, lipomas, liposarcomas, fat containing oncocytoma and xanthogranulomatous pyelonephritus.

AML are usually well defined but do not have a discrete capsule. They are often eccentrically located in the kidney and bulge out into the perinephric fat, although true local invasion is rare. Due to the haemangiomatous vascular component they usually enhance post IV contrast. On ultrasound AML are usually hyperechoic (bright) compared to the surrounding renal tissue. Non-contrast CT demonstrates a well-marginated cortical heterogeneous soft tissue lesion, containing fat. The identification of fat within the lesion will help differentiate renal carcinoma from AML as fat is rarely seen in renal cell carcinoma. However, approximately 5% of AMLs do not contain fat, which then makes differentiating from renal cell carcinoma difficult.

AML can either occur in isolation, not associated with another disease process, or in association with tuberous sclerosis (TS). A key ratio to remember for AML is 80:20. Eighty percent of AML are sporadic with a marked female predilection and usually single. Only 20% of AML are associated with TS; however 80% of people with TS have AML, often multiple and bilateral with an equal male to female ratio. If multiple and bilateral AML are seen, then other features of TS should be looked for (brain: cortical tubers, white matter abnormalities, subependymal nodules, giant cell astrocytoma; eyes: retinal hamartomas; heart: rhabdomyoma, lungs: approximately 1% of patients with TS will have lymphangioleiomyomatosis). Angiomyolipomas also occur in women with lymphangioleiomyomatosis, which has many pathophysiological similarities with TS.

The majority of people with AML are asymptomatic so most are discovered incidentally. If symptomatic, presentation can be with pain, local pressure effect (tumours can reach 20 cm) or bleeding, either haematuria or retroperitoneal haemorrhage. The main risk factor for bleeding is increasing size. Small tumours (less than 4 cm) have lower risk of bleeding and tend to grow slowly. Over 4 cm, the risk of bleeding is higher and pre-emptive treatment with selective embolization or partial nephrectomy may be offered. It is important to minimize the loss of functional renal parenchyma particularly in TS patients who often have multiple renal lesions. For this reason embolization is usually the preferred option, particularly in the presence of acute bleeding. Embolization is not 'curative', i.e. they do not involute completely and will often start to increase in size and vascularity again. For this reason complete infarction is not the aim, and particle or alcohol embolization with the aim of reducing tumoural vascularity is the preferred method. This allows further embolization treatment if required in the future which is not possible if the main feeding vessel is occluded with coils (alternative method). Surgical resection is usually reserved for atypical or rapidly enlarging lesions where the diagnosis is in doubt. Percutaneous biopsy of doubtful lesions is growing in popularity although there is a theoretical risk of tumour seeding along the biopsy track in malignant lesions. Small tumours are treated conservatively and usually followed up with serial ultrasound or MRI particularly if multiple. AML are heterogeneous on T2-weighted sequences.

CT is usually avoided for follow-up to reduce radiation burden, but is the initial investigation of choice if acute bleeding is suspected.

References

Evans JC, Curtis J. The radiological appearances of tuberous sclerosis. *Br J Radiol* 2000; **73**: 91–8.

Kenney PJ. Renal imaging. *Radiol Clin N Am* 2003; **41**(5): 1053–65.

Nawaz Khan A. *Angiomyolipoma, kidney*. May 2007. Available at: http://www.emedicine.com/radio/TOPIC28.HTM

Wagner BJ, Usaf M, Wong-You-Cheong JJ, Davis CJ. From the archives of the AFIP adult renal hamartomas. *RadioGraphics* 1997; **17**: 155–69.

Packet 5 Case 6 Question

INDRAN DAVAGNANAM

Clinical presentation

A 3-month-old baby presents with heart failure. A pre-treatment MRI is performed.

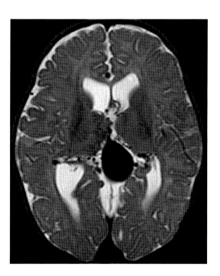

Figure 5.6.1

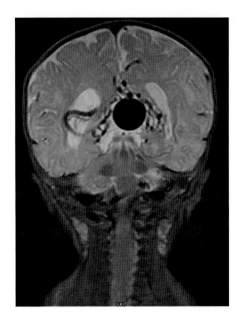

Figure 5.6.2

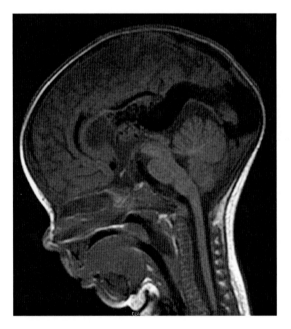

Figure 5.6.3

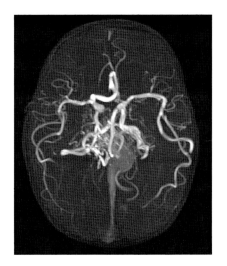

Figure 5.6.4

Packet 5 Case 6 Answer

Model answer

Examination
Non-contrast MRI brain and MR angiography of the circle of Willis (time of flight).

Findings
Axial and coronal T2-weighted images (Figures 5.6.1 and 5.6.2) demonstrate a midline posterior incisural hypointense mass (signal void) with some mass effect on the adjacent structures. Enlarged tortuous vessels are seen surrounding the described lesion. There is dilatation of the lateral ventricles.

Sagittal T1-weighted image (Figure 5.6.3) showing a hypointense (flow void) serpiginous structure along the line of the vein of Galen and superior straight sinus extending and involving the posterior aspect of the superior sagittal sinus and torcular herophili. Enlarged vessels are again identified in the proximity of this abnormality. There is inferior displacement of the tectal plate and narrowing of the cerebral aqueduct.

Single image from a maximal intensity projection (MIP) MRA (Figure 5.6.4) demonstrating signal within the described structure through to the straight sinus and torcular as well as through the numerous tortuous vessels surrounding it. Ectasia of the other arteries is also noted.

Interpretations
- Marked dilatation of the vein of Galen, embryonic falcine sinus, the posterior aspect of the superior sagittal sinus, torcular herophili and intracranial arteries.
- Dilatation and tortuosity of the vessels surrounding the vein of Galen (likely feeding arteries and arterialized veins).
- Compression of the tectal plate and narrowing of the cerebral aqueduct contributing to hydrocephalus.

Diagnosis
Vein of Galen malformation (VGM) with hydrocephalus.

Management

Likely to be under the care of paediatricians already for cardiac failure, but neuro-vascular surgeons need to be aware.

Cardiac failure treatment

Diagnostic digital subtracted angiography with a view to endovascular treatment.

Vein Of Galen aneurysmal malformations

Vein of Galen aneurysmal malformations (VGAMs) are rare congenital vascular malformations and are the commonest fetal vascular malformations representing 30% of all paediatric CNS vascular malformations. VGAMs are specific vascular malformations: a choroidal malformation and separate from an arteriovenous malformation draining into the vein of Galen (vein of Galen aneurysmal dilatation) and a vein of Galen varix. A vein of Galen varix is a varicose dilatation without any arteriovenous shunts.

VGAM occurs when a choroidal artery drains into the median vein of the prosencephalon, which is the embryonic vein of Galen. There is no venous connection to the deep venous system.

The malformation results from an intrauterine arteriovenous fistula developing at 6–11 weeks' gestation. It is the commonest extracardiac cause of high-output cardiac failure. Aortic coarctation and atrial septal defects are the commonest cardiac anomalies reported with VGAMs.

These malformations are classified into: (1) 'choroidal' type, with multiple shunting points and an unobstructed venous drainage; and (2) 'mural' type with one or few shunts and venous restriction. The development of hydrocephalus is secondary to venous hypertension and may be contributed to by narrowing of the cerebral aqueduct causing non-communicating hydrocephalus.

Patients present in one of three ways: in the neonatal period with extracardiac high-output cardiac failure, as an infant with symptoms of hydrocephalus and/or seizures or as an adolescent or young adult with haemorrhage. The degree of the arteriovenous shunt is variable and is a factor in determining at what age the child may present clinically.

Cardiac failure was the most common cause of death in these patients before the advent of endovascular treatment. Endovascular embolization treatment of the shunting is the preferred therapy in order to decrease the severity of cardiac failure and to preserve neurological function. This occurs in conjunction with aggressive medical treatment of the cardiac failure. However, endovascular embolization carries significant risks: aneurysm perforation, cerebral infarction and distant migration of emboli.

VGAM may be suggested with antenatal ultrasound especially if there is severe heart failure in utero, which can present as polyhydramnios or hydrops fetalis.

Further imaging with ante- and postnatal fetal MR is essential to characterization and assess treatment options, complications relating to the VGM (hydrocephalus or ischaemic brain injury), parental counselling and prognosis. On MR imaging, VGAM is seen as a large midline signal void on T2-weighted sequences. If feeding vessels are present, they are seen as serpiginous signal voids related to the midline VGAM.

References

Alvarez H, Monaco RG, Rodesch G et al. Vein of Galen aneurysmal malformations. *Neuroimag Clin N Am* 2007; **17**: 189–206.

Atlas SW. *Magnetic resonance imaging of the brain and spine*, Vol I, 4th edn. Lippincott, Williams & Wilkins; 2008: 260–2.

Barkovich AJ. *Pediatric neuroimaging*, 4th ed. Philadephia: Lippincott, Williams & Wilkins; 2005: 875–84.

Epelman M, Daneman A, Blaser SI et al. Differential diagnosis of intracranial cystic lesions at head ultrasound: correlation with CT and MR imaging. *RadioGraphics* 2006; **26**: 173–96.

Golja AM, Estroff JA, Robertson RL. Fetal imaging of central nervous system abnormalities. *Neuroimag Clin N Am* 2004; **14**: 293–306.

McElhinney DB, Halbach VV, Silverman NH, Dowd CF, Hanley FL. Congenital cardiac anomalies with vein of Galen malformations in infants. *Arch Dis Child* 1998; **78**: 548–51.

Osborn A, Blasen S, Salzman K et al. *Diagnostic imaging: brain*, 1st ed. Amirsys/Elsevier; 2004 I; **5**: 12–15.

Packet 6 Case 1 Question

KIAT TAN

Clinical history

A 45-year-old lady presents with a history of chronic non-specific episodes of severe abdominal pain and nausea and vomiting. Plain radiography, ultrasound, barium studies and endoscopy have all been reported as normal.

(a)

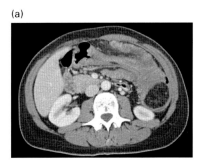

(b)

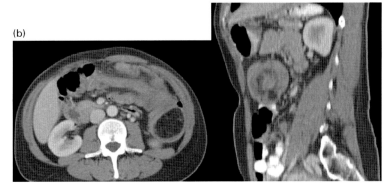

Figure 6.1.1a, b

Packet 6 Case 1 Answer

Model answer

Examination
CT scan of the abdomen and pelvis with IV and oral contrast.

Findings and interpretations
- Smooth lesion with a diameter of around 4 cm of fat attenuation in the small bowel, which has a targetoid appearance on the sagittal image.
- No evidence of large or small bowel dilatation.
- No free gas or free fluid seen.

Diagnosis
Intussusception of the small bowel. This is most likely to be due to a lipoma.
   The presence of liposarcoma is extremely unlikely but this cannot be ruled out.

Management
The case needs to be discussed with surgeons with a view to surgical removal and reduction. The intussusception may compromise the blood supply resulting in ischaemic and necrotic bowel.

Small bowel lipoma

Intussusception is very uncommon in adults and is more commonly seen in the paediatric population. Adult cases account for approximately 5% of all intussusception cases; 1% are the cause of all bowel obstruction cases and 0.003%–0.02% of all hospital admissions. Intussusception occurs when a proximal segment of bowel, termed the intussusceptum, invaginates into the lumen of the adjacent distal bowel segment, termed intussuscipiens. It can occur anywhere in the bowel and can be between either segments of large bowel (colo-colic), large–small bowel (ileo-colic) or small bowel–small bowel (ileo-ileal). In adults the clinical presentation differs; patients may present with acute, intermittent or chronic pain and obstruction. Other symptoms include nausea, vomiting, fever, diarrhoea and abdominal pain. They can often be misdiagnosed initially.

Small bowel intussusception is most often due to a tumour. The lead point in adults is commonly due to tumour whilst in children it is most often enlarged lymph nodes or hyperplastic lymphoid tissue. Malignancy in adults needs to be excluded primarily; it has been estimated that 20–50% of cases in adults are due to a malignancy.

Small bowel lipomas are the second most common benign tumours of the small bowel, second only to leiomyomas. Small bowel lipomas are most often unifocal but can be multiple. Like leiomyomas, these lesions are submucosal and can project into the lumen, potentially causing intussusception.

Ultrasound is helpful in diagnosis especially in the paediatric population, and is usually an appropriate initial investigation after plain radiography to interrogate the bowel for a possible intussusception. The typical ultrasound features of an intussusception have been described as a 'pseudokidney' or a 'target' appearance. The optical illusion of a pseudokidney is described because the intussusceptum is the centre and the oedematous intussuscipiens forms the external ring forming an image of a pseudokidney on ultrasound. There is however a potential limitation: ultrasound is of limited value in acute intestinal obstruction due to abundant overlying bowel gas shadows. CT is the preferred imaging modality in a patient with acute abdominal obstruction and in adults, as in this case. CT will delineate any complications associated with the intussusception, especially if the cause is due to a malignant process. Surgical intervention is necessary in adults whatever the cause. In cases due to benign pathology, lesions may require resection to prevent recurrence.

References

Azar T, Berger DL. Review article: adult intussusception. *Ann Surg* 1997; **226**(2): 134–8.

Meshikhes A-WN, Al-Momen SAM, Fayiza TAT, Al-Jaroof1 AH. Adult intussusception caused by a lipoma in the small bowel: report of a case. *Surgery Today* 2005; **35**(2): 1436–2813.

Oyen TL, Wolthuis AM, Tollens T, Aelvoet C, Vanrijkel JP. Ileo-ileal intussusception secondary to a lipoma: a literature review. *Acta Chir Belg* 2007; **107**: 60–3.

Uysal S, Tuncbilek I, Gokharman D et al. Visualization of fat in the intussusception: lipoma or mesenteric adipose tissue? *Eur J Radiol* 2006; **57**: 81–3.

Packet 6 Case 2 Question

MANDY WILLIAMS

Clinical history

A 68-year-old woman presents with thoracic back pain, worse at night. There is a previous history of breast cancer 5 years ago. No history of recent trauma.

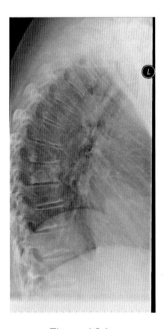

Figure 6.2.1

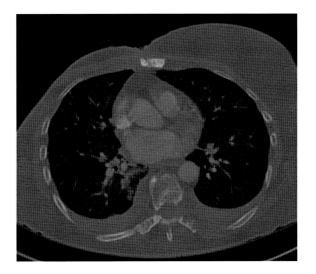

Figure 6.2.2

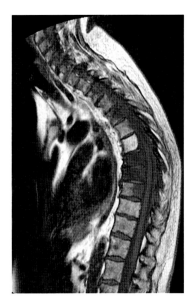

Figure 6.2.3

Packet 6 Case 2 Answer

Model answer

Examination
- Lateral radiograph of the thoracic spine (Figure 6.2.1).
- CT thorax on bone windows (Figure 6.2.2).
- T1-weighted MRI of the thoracic spine (Figure 6.2.3).

Findings and interpretations

Plain radiograph
- There is sclerosis of a mid thoracic vertebral body that extends into the pedicle. There is loss of vertebral body height. The vertebral body superior to it also shows areas of sclerosis in its posterior aspect.
- The cortex is ill defined and there is evidence of bone destruction.
- The appearances would be consistent with multiple sclerotic metastases from breast carcinoma.

MRI thoracic spine
- There are multiple areas of low signal intensites in a number of the thoracic vertebral bodies on T1-weighted imaging. The anterior and posterior elements are involved which is highly suspicious of a malignant process. Benign bone lesions usually involve the anterior elements only.
- On these sagittal sequences the spinal cord does not appear compressed; however axial images would be needed to confirm this.
- The sclerotic areas on plain film correspond to the low signal on T1-weighted MRI sequence. The fatty bone marrow usually demonstrates high signal on T1-weighted imaging but appears replaced with tumour hence the low signal on the T1-weighted sequence.

Diagnosis
In this clinical context, this most probably represents multiple metastases from the past history of breast carcinoma.

Differential diagnosis
- Lymphoma.
- Lytic metastases post radiotherapy/chemotherapy.

- Multiple myeloma – they are sclerotic in 3%.
- Bone infarcts and this is an unusual site.
- (In a male patient the most likely primary would be prostatic carcinoma.)

Management
The entire spine should be imaged with MRI axial and sagittal T1-weighted, T2-weighted and sagittal STIR assessing for cord compression and disease extent. If the cord is compressed urgent radiotherapy and/or surgical decompression may be needed. This needs to be communicated to the referring clinican.

The remainder of the skeleton can be imaged with a 99mTc MDP bone scan.

Skeletal metastases

The imaging features of skeletal metastases are well described. The MR features of marrow changes in relation to skeletal metastases will be discussed.

Plain radiograph
- Bone destruction that typically involves the posterior elements.
- Bony scleroses or lytic areas; dependent upon the primary carcinoma involved.
  (A comprehensive list can be obtained from *Aids to radiological differential diagnosis*).
- There can be loss of vertebral body height from pathological fractures and collapse.
- Multiple bones are involved.

Nuclear medicine
- Increased uptake of radiotracer in multiple areas.
- Plain radiographic changes in the same areas of increased uptake on bone scan.

CT
High-resolution CT with bony reconstruction should be used. Multiplanar reconstruction is very helpful; as an example, rib lesions appear more conspicuous on the sagittal reformats.

Metastases appear as areas of bone destruction. The cortex is ill defined and there may be an associated soft tissue mass (see Figure 6.2.2).

MR imaging of marrow infiltration
The bone marrow signal in the vertebral column is dependent upon the age of the patient. Normal marrow consists of red and yellow elements within the bony trabecular network of the vertebral body. The red marrow represents haemopoietic areas whilst the function of the yellow marrow is not well understood but is thought to represent inactive haemopoietic tissue (presumed 'fatty marrow'), which increases in its distribution as we age. Re-conversion can occur from yellow to red, in certain states, such as anaemia from any cause (aplastic anaemia, high altitude, smoking, chronic airways disease).

There is no doubt that MRI tends to be better at detecting metastases in the spine and pelvis as compared to scintigraphy. Marrow signal is also affected by other processes: infection, inflammatory including post-radiotherapy changes and metabolic disorders.

Red marrow signal
- Slightly higher signal on T1-weighted sequences (compared to skeletal muscle signal).

Yellow marrow signal
- High on T1- and T2-weighted sequences.
- Follows the signal of fat on all imaging sequences.
- Haemangioma follows the signal of fat and is well circumscribed.

In metastatic disease the usual standard sequence protocol consists of sagittal and axial T1- and T2-weighted and short tau inversion recovery (STIR)/fat saturation sequences. These sequences highlight the differences between normal fatty bone marrow and bone infiltrated with tumour. T2-weighted sequences will show areas of high signal if there are areas of associated bone oedema. STIR and fat saturation sequences will show areas of high signal in infiltrated bone as it fully suppresses the yellow ('fat') marrow signal. Normal marrow on STIR sequence results in a uniformly low signal. Red marrow on STIR sequence demonstrates a slightly increased signal compared to muscle.

T1-weighted sequence with fat saturation and post-contrast studies can be used instead of STIR depending on institutional preference.

Metastatic disease
- Usually low on T1-weighted sequence compared with muscle signal.
- High on T2-weighted sequence.
- Usually enhances with IV contrast.
- Multifocal ± discontinuous depending on disease extent.
- Involvement of the pedicle (posterior elements).
- Presence of an epidural mass.
- Sclerotic metastases (most often breast or prostatic carcinoma) – often low on T1- and T2-weighting.

Multiple myeloma affecting the marrow will be mentioned briefly as it has a different signal pattern compared to other spinal metastases and is not an uncommon disease entity.
It can produce:

- Diffuse marrow abnormality (commonly in patients with severe disease).
- Marrow signal may be normal.
- Focal lesions, which are well defined.
- Variegated pattern.

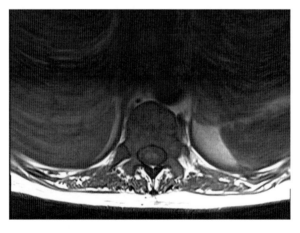

Figure 6.2.4 Myeloma. Axial T1-weighted image of the thoracic spine. The normal marrow signal is replaced by low T1-weighted signal representing tumour involving all the elements of the spine.

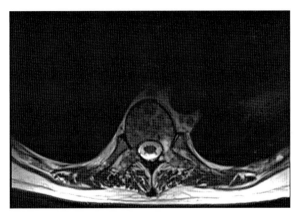

Figure 6.2.5 Myeloma. Axial T2-weighted image of the thoracic spine. The normal marrow signal is replaced by heterogeneous T2-weighted signal representing tumour. There is involvement of both the anterior and posterior columns.

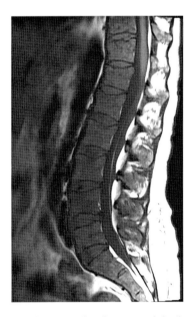

Figure 6.2.6 Myeloma. Sagittal T1-weighted image of the lumbar spine. Diffuse involvement of the spine is demonstrated.

Post treatment for multiple myeloma, the T2-weighted signal may change (decreases) or there is reduced enhancement in response to treatment.

Figures 6.2.4 to 6.2.7 are from a patient with known clinical diagnosis of multiple myeloma.

References

Chapman S, Nakielny R. *Aids to radiological differential diagnosis*, 5th ed. Edinburgh: Saunders; 2003.

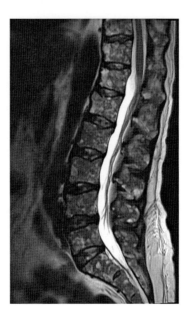

Figure 6.2.7 Myeloma. Sagittal T2-weighted image of the lumbar spine.

Nelson E, Eustace SJ. Whole body magnetic resonance imaging: a valuable adjunct to clinical examination. *BMJ* 2004; **328**: 1387–8.

Tall MA, Thompson AK, Vertinsky T, Palka PS. MR Imaging of the spinal bone marrow. *Magn Reson Imaging Clin N Am* 2007; **15**: 175–98.

Vanel D. MRI of bone metastases: choice of sequences. *Cancer Imag* 2004; **4**(1): 30–5.

Packet 6 Case 3 Question

NEIL COLLIN

Clinical history

A 41-year-old male presents with worsening shortness of breath.

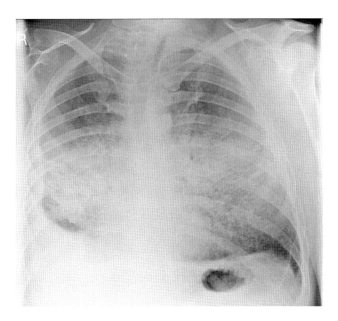

Figure 6.3.1

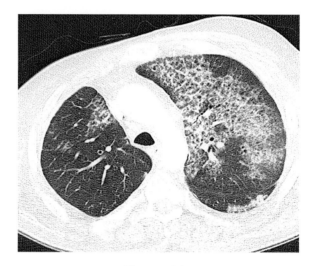

Figure 6.3.2

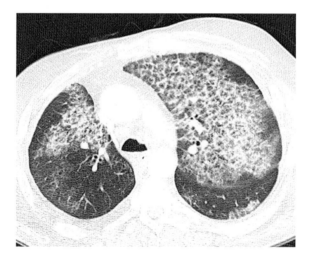

Figure 6.3.3

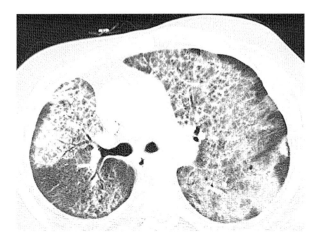

Figure 6.3.4

Packet 6 Case 3 Answer

Model answer

Examinations
- Frontal chest radiograph (Figure 6.3.1).
- Axial images from a high-resolution CT (HRCT) (Figures 6.3.2 to 6.3.4).

Findings and interpretations

Frontal chest radiograph
- Bilateral perihilar abnormality, mixed nodular airspace and reticular opacification.
- Blunting of right costophrenic angle consistent with small right pleural effusion.
- Heart size is difficult to assess but appears grossly normal.
- Normal upper zone vascular markings.
- Bones normal.

HRCT chest
- Patchy ground glass opacification.
- Thickening of interlobular and intralobular septa.
- Lung apices spared, with relatively normal lung parenchyma.
- Normal upper zone vascularity.

Diagnosis
Pulmonary alveolar proteinosis.

Differential diagnosis
- Pulmonary oedema/ARDS.
- Sarcoid.
- Alveolar cell carcinoma.
- Atypical infections.

Management
Refer to chest physician for bronchoscopy ± lavage, and further investigation to rule out underlying cause.

Pulmonary alveolar proteinosis

Pulmonary alveolar proteinosis (PAP) is a rare lung disease, with an incidence of approximately 0.36 per 100 000 people. There are three distinct subgroups of PAP: idiopathic (other terminology include acquired, or adult type), secondary and congenital form.

The acquired form comprises greater than 90% of all cases with no cause identified. Patients are usually affected in their fifth decade and three-quarters of these will have a history of smoking. In this group of smokers, men are affected more frequently than women whilst there is no gender bias in the non-smoker subset.

The secondary form is seen in patients with inhalation exposure to silica, cement dust, aluminium dust, titanium dioxide, nitrogen dioxide, fibreglass exposure, underlying haematological malignancy and immunosuppressive disorders.

In PAP the alveoli fill with an excess of pulmonary surfactant produced by type II pneumocytes. There appears to be a dysfunction in surfactant proteins or impaired function of granulocyte-macrophage colony-simulating factor (GM-CSF) in the inherited subgroup.

Clinical presentation is insidious with gradual onset of shortness of breath the most consistent feature. Other clinical symptoms include a dry cough, fatigue, chest pain, weight loss and haemoptysis.

Radiographic signs may pre-date onset of clinical symptoms in up to a third of patients.

Initially the chest radiograph findings are abnormal and non-specific. The CXR findings may resemble non-cardiogenic pulmonary oedema, with bilateral perihilar 'bat's-wing' nodular opacities coalescing into consolidation and sparing of the costophrenic angles and apices. The findings are usually symmetrical but may occasionally be unilateral. Cardiomegaly and pleural effusions are not normally present, pulmonary vascularity is normal, and lymphadenopathy is rare.

What is also striking is the contrast in the dramatic radiological findings and modest clinical symptoms.

Although there is some associated inflammatory response, this does not often progress to widespread pulmonary fibrosis.

HRCT of the chest shows areas of patchy ground-glass opacification with smooth interlobular septal thickening, which produces a pattern known as 'crazy paving'. The crazy paving pattern is described as being well-defined bilateral areas with a widespread geographical distribution. Normal appearing lung parenchyma is interposed between the areas of abnormality. There is no zonal predominance for the crazy paving pattern. Crazy paving is seen in other diseases and the differential includes: pulmonary oedema (cardiac failure), infection (various and includes pneumocystis pneumonia), granulomatous disease (sarcoidosis), neoplastic disease (lymphangitic carinomatosis and alveolar cell carcinoma), hypersensitivity pneumonitis and acute respiratory distress syndrome (ARDS).

The definitive diagnosis for PAP is bronchoalveolar lavage and positive staining for periodic acid-Schiff stain.

Treatment for idiopathic PAP consists of repeated treatments of whole lung bronchial lavage to wash out the excess surfactant. Reports of prognosis are varied, ranging from 30% mortality to spontaneous recovery. Treated survival is over 90% although recurrence may require further treatment.

Congenital PAP will require lung transplantation and secondary PAP requires environmental modification.

A final but significant point to remember is that PAP occurs in smokers; the presence of a concurrent lung carcinoma related to smoking rather than PAP has been reported and should be borne in mind.

In this case there was previous history of trauma to the right side of the chest, which accounts for the reduced volume of the right hemi-thorax.

References

Frazier AA, Franks TJ, Cooke E et al. From the Archives of AFIP: Pulmonary alveolar proteinosis. *RadioGraphics* 2008; **28**(3): 883–99.

Gotway MB, Theodore JL. *Alveolar proteinosis*. Updated 30 Dec 2008. Available at: http://emedicine.medscape.com/article/352741-overview

Shah PL, Hansell D, Lawson PR et al. Pulmonary alveolar proteinosis: clinical aspects and current concepts on pathogenesis. *Thorax* 2000; **55**(1): 67–77.

Packet 6 Case 4 Question

INDRAN DAVAGNANAM

Clinical history

A child presents with worsening headaches age 7 (Figures 6.4.1–6.4.3). There is a history of seizures and delayed milestones age 3 (Figures 6.4.4–6.4.5).

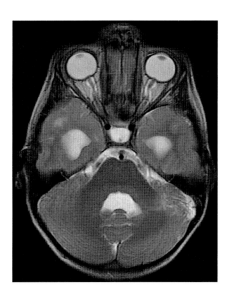

Figure 6.4.1

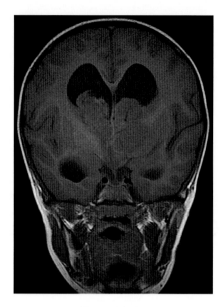

Figure 6.4.2

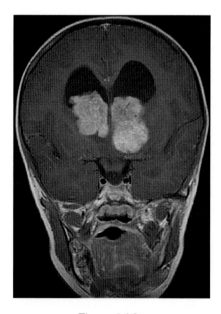

Figure 6.4.3

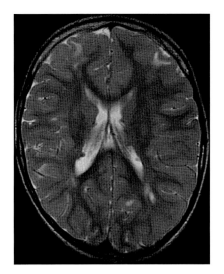

Figure 6.4.4

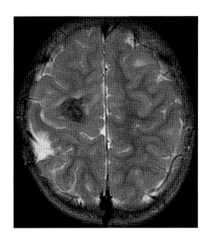

Figure 6.4.5

Packet 6 Case 4 Answer

Model answer

Examination
Pre- and post-contrast MRI brain.

Findings

MRI brain (age 7)
- Axial T2-weighted image showing dilatation of the temporal horns of the lateral ventricles. Expansion of the optic sheaths with adjacent high T2 signal paralleling the optic nerve. There is bulging of the optic nerve heads into the globes (Figure 6.4.1).
- Coronal T1-weighted pre-contrast image demonstrates bilateral intraventricular large masses at the level of the foramen of Monro. There is dilatation of the lateral ventricles and effacement of the cortical sulci (Figure 6.4.2).
- Coronal T1-weighted post-contrast image demonstrates bilateral avid enhancement of the described masses at the foramina of Monro (Figure 6.4.3).

MRI brain (age 3)
- Axial T2-weighted image demonstrates subependymal low signal nodules, bifrontal, left parietal subcortical and deep white matter T2-weighted high signal foci (Figure 6.4.4).
- Axial T2-weighted image demonstrates a right posterior frontal cortical or subcortical lesion (difficult to be certain on the limited imaging) and marked low signal (Figure 6.4.5).

Interpretations
- Multiple subependymal hamartomas.
- Multiple cortical tubers.
- There is calcification of the tuber in the right superior frontal gyrus.
- Bilateral large subependymal masses compatible with giant cell astrocytomas.
- Obstructive hydrocephalus and papilloedema (Figure 6.4.1).

Diagnosis
Tuberous sclerosis (TS) with bilateral large subependymal giant cell astrocytomas causing obstructive hydrocephalus.

Management

The findings are compatible with an acute presentation and the on-call or referring clinical team needs to be contacted to communicate the urgent neurosurgical assessment and input.

Once stabilized and on subsequent follow-up, further imaging of the abdominal viscera, lungs and heart is most likely required to assess for multisystem involvement.

Tuberous sclerosis (TS)

Desire-Magloire Bourneville described the pathology and neurological manifestations of TS in 1880, which is eponymously known as Bourneville disease. It is an inherited autosomal dominant neurocutaneous disorder that involves multiple organ systems. There is variability in its expression even within the same family. MR is very valuable in screening family members where clinical markers may not be apparent and in cases where the CT may be normal. Genetic research has yielded the identification of the TSC1 gene on chromosome 9 and TSC2 gene on chromosome 16. Classically, TS has been characterized by the clinical triad of mental retardation (half of the affected population), epilepsy (cortical tubers) and skin lesions; facial angiofibromas misconceived as adenoma sebaceum by dermatologists in the 1890s. Angiofibromas usually start before puberty and in the nasolabial fold, spreading across the face in a malar distribution.

Neuroimaging plays a role in the diagnosis with characteristic abnormalities in 95% of affected patients on imaging at birth, preceding the cutaneous manifestations. The clinical significance is highly important given the nature of the autosomal dominant inheritance pattern. This enables genetic counselling along with follow-up and monitoring of CNS and non-CNS lesions, which have a propensity to degenerate or become haemorrhagic.

Retinal hamartomas form the commonest of the ocular findings and can provide clinical markers for initial diagnosis.

Several characteristic lesions occur in the brain. The most common of the intracranial features are the subependymal hamartomas which are histologically distinct from cortical hamartomas (tubers). The subependymal nodules tend to be located along the ventricular surface of the caudate nucleus, immediately posterior to the foramen of Monro (in the caudothalamic groove). These rarely calcify in the first year of life, but increasingly do so as the patient ages and show variable post-contrast enhancement. Subependymal nodules in TS have the same signal as grey matter on MR imaging. They can be differentiated from heterotopic grey matter subependymal nodules due to the difference in orientation along the subependymal ventricular margin. Heterotopic grey matter does not calcify. The subependymal nodules of TS enhance on MR; this is an expected finding and does not indicate malignant transformation.

Subependymal giant cell astrocytoma is a low-grade tumour (classification World Health Organization grade 1). They represent enlarging subependymal nodules, usually situated near the foramina of Monro. These are distinct from subependymal nodules by virtue of their size and tendency to enlarge, usually resulting in the clinical presentation of hydrocephalus. Subependymal nodules are usually less than 15 mm in diameter.

Cerebral hamartomas are most commonly supratentorial, with 8%–15% of affected patients having cerebellar tubers. Calcification of these increases with age; 50% of patients with TS have calcified tubers by the age of 10. On CT cortical hamartomas appear as cortical lucencies within broadened gyri and are difficult to distinguish in adults if non-calcified. On MRI they are similar in signal intensity to subependymal hamartomas in both unmyelinated and mature brains, but are most conspicuous on FLAIR sequences. Non-cortical-based islets of groupings of giant neurones, dysplastic glial and neuronal cells as well as hypomyelination, also appear as T2-weighted white matter bright lesions on MR in TS.

Non-CNS manifestations include angiomyolipomas, benign rhabdomyomas of the heart (single or multiple), pulmonary lymphangioleiomyomatosis (in only 1% of patients with TS), adenomas and lipomas of the abdominal viscera, renal hamartomas, bone cysts of the cranium, metacarpals and phalanges, as well as aneurysms. Other major features include ungul or periungual fibroma and classical shagreen patch naevi.

Current recommendations are for cranial imaging every 1–3 years in children and renal ultrasound every 1–3 years at all ages.

References

Atlas SW. *Magnetic resonance imaging of the brain and spine*, 4th ed. Philadelphia: Lippincott, Williams & Wilkins; Volume **I;II** 0000: 389–98.

Barkovich AJ. *Pediatric neuroimaging*, 4th ed. Philadelphia: Lippincott, Williams & Wilkins; 2005: 463–76.

Evans JC, Curtis J. The radiological appearance of tuberous sclerosis. *Br J Radiol* 2000; **73**: 91–8.

McMurdo K, Moore SG, Brant-Zawadzki M et al. MR imaging of intracranial tuberous sclerosis. *AJR* 1987; **148**: 791–6.

Morse RP. Tuberous sclerosis. *Arch Neurol* 1998; **55**: 1257–8.

Northrup H, Wheless JW, Bertin TK, Lewis RA. Variability of expression in tuberous sclerosis. *J Med Genet* 1993; **30**: 41–3.

Smirniotopoulous JG. Neuroimaging of phakomatoses. *Neuroimag Clin N Am* 2004; **14**: 171–83.

Packet 6 Case 5 Question

KATE TAYLOR-ROBINSON

Clinical history

A 1-year-old baby presents with vomiting and abdominal distension.

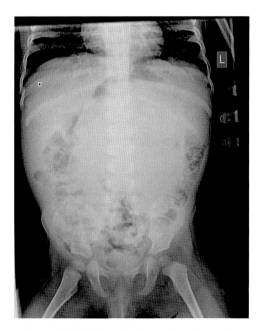

Figure 6.5.1 Plain abdominal radiograph.

(a)

(b)

(c)

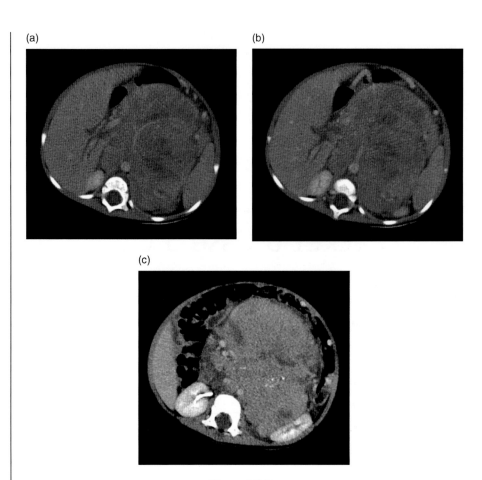

Figure 6.5.2

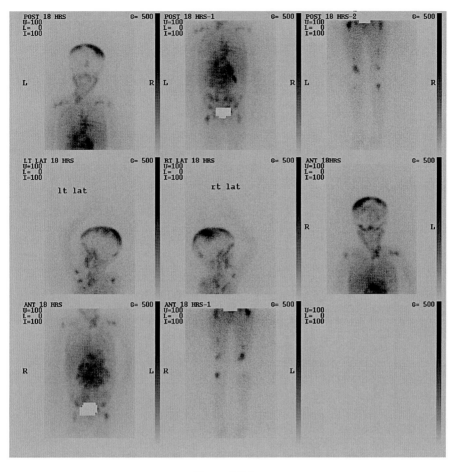

Figure 6.5.3

Packet 6 Case 5 Answer

Model answer

Examination
- Plain abdominal radiograph (Figure 6.5.1).
- Selected images from a contrast-enhanced CT abdomen and pelvis (Figures 6.5.2a–c).
- Metaiodobenzylguanidine (MIBG) scan (Figure 6.5.3).

Findings and interpretations
The plain radiograph demonstrates a large soft tissue mass occupying the centre of the abdomen displacing surrounding bowel gas. No calcification is evident on plain film.

CT demonstrates a large soft tissue mass centred in the region of the left adrenal gland with areas of calcification and cystic degeneration. The coeliac axis is completely engulfed and stretched by the mass. Lobular contour in the right para-aortic region suggests spread to local lymph nodes. No liver metastases are demonstrated on these slices. The kidneys appear separate from the mass and appear to be excreting contrast normally with no hydronephrosis.

The MIBG scan demonstrates avid tracer uptake by the known abdominal mass. There is also evidence of widespread skeletal metastasis including foci in the calvarium, scapulae, femora, right tibia, spine and pelvis. Normal uptake is noted in the salivary glands, heart, liver and bladder.

Diagnosis
Metastatic neuroblastoma stage 4.

Differential diagnosis
Wilms' tumour may produce a large abdominal mass in young children. However, it tends to occur in an older age group, is less likely to be calcified, is more likely to displace the vessels and usually demonstrates the claw sign demonstrating its origin from the kidney. It does not take up MIBG, unlike neuroblastoma.

Management
- Examine the remaining images for signs of spinal canal invasion – consider MRI if CT equivocal.

- Perform 99mTc MDP bone scan to further demonstrate the extent of skeletal involvement.
- Consider image-guided biopsy for tissue diagnosis.
- Refer urgently to paediatric oncology multidisciplinary team.

Neuroblastoma

Peripheral neuroblastic tumours are a heterogenous group of tumours, which belong to the 'small blue round cell' tumours of childhood. They include the Ewing family of tumours, lymphoma and neuroblastic tumours.

Neuroblastic histopathological subtypes are neuroblastomas, ganglioneuroblastoma and ganglioneuroma. Neuroblastoma is the most undifferentiated from these three subtypes.

Neuroblastoma is the most common extracranial solid malignancy in children, accounting for approximately 8–10% of all childhood cancers. They can occur anywhere along the sympathetic chain from cells of neural crest origin.

Clinical presentation depends on the site of origin, but for the greater part, the abdomen is a common site; 35% arise from the adrenal medulla and another 35% arise from the extra-adrenal retro-peritoneum (para-vertebral sympathetic ganglia). Other less common sites of involvement (in descending order of frequency) are the posterior mediastinum, pelvis and neck. The peak age is 2 years, most children present between the ages of 1 and 5. There is no particular race or worldwide geographical predilection but there is a minor increase in frequency in males compared to females (ratio of 1.2:1). There has not been a consistent genetic abnormality identified to date, and it is known that a rare familial form exists with the child presenting at a younger age and involvement with multiple sites. It can also occur in disorders of neural crest cell origin; neurofibromatosis 1 and Hirschsprung disease, however no specific genetic link has been identified.

Diagnosis requires either biopsy material or neuroblastoma cells in a bone marrow sample with raised urinary or serum catecholamine/metabolites. Histologically the tumour cannot be distinguished from other 'small blue round cell' tumours by the usual haematoxylin-eosin stain and requires immunohistochemical assessment for positive neural markers and negative staining for other 'small blue round cell' markers.

In this disease entity, imaging can help assess surgical resectability and metastatic spread. These factors will aid treatment options and prognostic stratification.

Initial imaging with CT and further evaluation with MRI should be considered if CT is equivocal or if neurological and spinal invasion is suggested clinically.

It is an invasive tumour with a tendency to engulf/encase rather than displace vessels, and a tendency to invade the spinal canal. Eighty percent have some calcification on CT. Invasion of the kidneys can mimic a Wilms' tumour. On MRI the tumour appears iso to low signal on T1-weighted and bright on T2-weighted with fat suppression and enhancement post-contrast. Calcification will show as signal void on T2-weighting or gradient echo sequences.

Disease spread is via the lymphatics and haematogenous route and thus the most common sites of metastases are to liver, bone and bone marrow. Age has been shown to be an important clinical prognostic factor and tends to be worse with increasing age. Children older than 1–2 years have worse prognosis than younger ones. In children it is worth considering neuroblastoma and lymphoma as the diagnosis when soft tissue displaces the abdominal aorta anteriorly.

Both the 99mTc MDP bone scan and I-123 MIBG scan are of use in staging neuroblastoma. Thirty percent of neuroblastomas are not MIBG avid. In some cases skeletal metastases, which are both cortical and medullary, are better shown on an MDP bone scan.

Anatomical stage depends on extension beyond organ of origin (stage 2, 75% survival), crossing the midline (stage 3) and distant metastases (stage 4, 10% survival). Interestingly, stage 4S in children under the age of 1 comprises metastatic disease confined to the skin, liver and bone marrow and has an excellent prognosis with minimal treatment.

References

Lane F. *Diagnostic imaging: pediatrics*, 1st ed. Amirsys Inc. Donnelly/Elsevier; 2005 **5**: 78–81.

Park JR, Eggert A, Caron H. Neuroblastoma: biology, prognosis and treatment. *Pediatr Clin N Am* 2008; **55**: 97–120.

Siegel MI, Jaju A. MR imaging of neuroblastic masses. *Magn Reson Imaging Clin N Am* 2008; **16**: 499–513.

Slovis TL. *Caffey's pediatric diagnostic imaging*, 11th ed. Mosby Elsevier; 2008: 2215–20.

Packet 6 Case 6 Question

MONICA KHANNA

Clinical history

A 33-year-old intravenous drug user presents with groin pain, back pain and fevers.

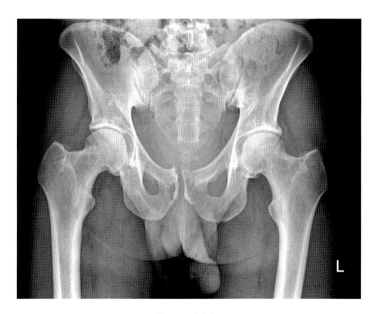

Figure 6.6.1

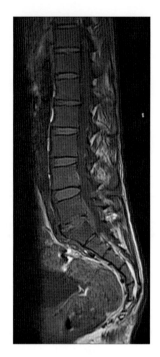

Figure 6.6.2

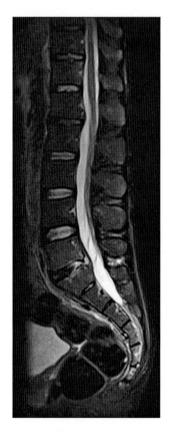

Figure 6.6.3

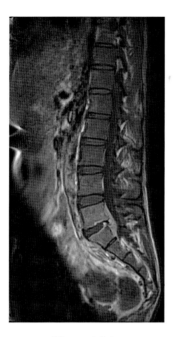

Figure 6.6.4

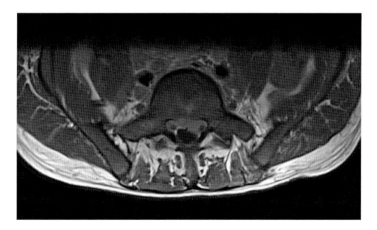

Figure 6.6.5

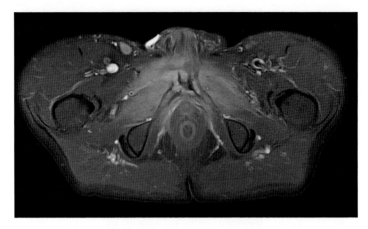

Figure 6.6.6

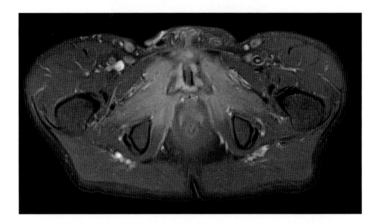

Figure 6.6.7

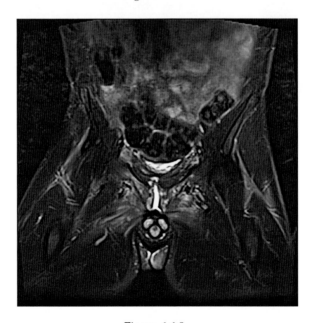

Figure 6.6.8

Answers to follow on page 228

Packet 6 Case 6 Answer

Model answer

Examination
- AP pelvic radiograph (Figure 6.6.1).
- Sagittal T1-weighted MR lumbar spine (Figure 6.6.2).
- Sagittal STIR MR lumbar spine (Figure 6.6.3).
- Sagittal T1-weighted and fat saturated post-contrast MR lumbar spine (Figure 6.6.4).
- Axial T1-weighted and fat saturated post-contrast MR lumbar spine (Figure 6.6.5).
- Axial T1-weighted and fat saturated post-contrast MR pubis (Figures 6.6.6 and 6.6.7).
- Coronal STIR MR pubis (Figure 6.6.8).

Findings and interpretations

AP pelvic radiograph
Widening of the symphysis pubis with joint margin irregularity and peri-articular lucency.

MR lumbar spine
T1-weighted lumbar spine images demonstrates a diffuse reduction in bone marrow signal, loss of disc height at L5/S1 level with irregularity and erosion of the posterior aspect of the end plates in association with epidural extension. Post contrast demonstrates there is subtle peripheral enhancement of the end plate erosions with diffuse enhancement of the epidural soft tissue extension consistent with a phlegmon. The epidural phlegmon is causing indentation on the anterior aspect of the theca and extends around both L5 nerve roots within the lateral recesses.

MR pubis
- There is high STIR signal within the pubic rami and fluid signal within the symphysis pubis joint.
- There is bone marrow enhancement within the pubic rami centred at the symphysis pubis with soft tissue extension on the right consistent with a phlegmon.
- There is extensive surrounding soft tissue high signal compatible with oedema within the adductor muscles bilaterally.

Diagnosis

Pyogenic discitis and associated epidural phlegmon at L5/S1.

Septic arthritis of the symphysis pubis joint with associated osteomyelitis within the pubic rami.

Differential diagnosis

Tuberculous discitis.

Management

- Diagnostic aspiration of joint/disc to obtain a sample for microbiology (causative organism), culture and sensitivity.
- Imaging of the whole spine to exclude involvement of other vertebral levels.
- Treatment with IV antibiotics with appropriate sensitivity.

Vertebral osteomyelitis

Osteomyelitis infection can be classified as due to either pyogenic or non-pyogenic (granulomatous) causes. Vertebral osteomyelitis is a disease process that can involve the bony and soft tissues of the neural axis and not just the vertebral body. The most common causative organisms are *Staphylococcus aureus*, *Streptococcus* and *Pneumococcus* in pyogenic osteomyelitis, the most common of these being *Staphylococcus aureus* (40–45%). *Mycobacterium tuberculosis* is the most common cause of granulomatous osteomyelitis. Distinguishing between pyogenic and tuberculous spondylodiscitis is difficult.

Routes of infection include haematogenous spread, or rarely contiguous spread from direct inoculation. The arterial route is thought to be more likely than via the venous system. The most common cause in pyogenic osteomyelitis is systemic bacteraemia, usually from a cutaneous, urinary or pulmonary infection. This occurred secondary to intravenous drug use in this case. Risk factors include immunosuppression, previous/recent surgery, indwelling catheters/lines, increasing age and intravenous drug use. There is a slight male predominance and adults are more commonly affected than children. More than 50% of cases occur in the 5th to 6th decade.

Tuberculous osteomyelitis should be considered if there is a previous history. Extra-pulmonary disease is a consideration in patients with pyrexia of unknown origin and immunosuppression/immunosuppressed states (chemotherapy, diabetics, chronic liver, chronic renal diseases and autoimmune disorders).

Clinically, vertebral osteomyelitis may present with back pain, night waking and fevers (pyrexia of unknown origin). The pain is continuous and does not disperse with rest or conservative treatment.

In adults, pyogenic infection typically begins in the subchondral portion of the vertebral body and subsequently spreads to the adjacent disc due to the same segmental arterial supply to both. The pattern of spread in tuberculous infection is to the adjacent vertebral body via the sub-ligamentous route. This means that spread occurs along the anterior and/or posterior longitudinal ligaments with relative sparing of the disc.

Children have richly vascularized intervertebral discs, which can become infected initially before spreading to the vertebral bodies.

Pyogenic spondylitis may occur anywhere in the spine, the order of frequency of occurrence being: lumbar (56%) followed by the thoracic spine (35%), cervical (up to 20%) and sacral region. In TB osteomyelitis the order of frequency is different: thoracic > lumbar > cervical.

It is important to remember that multifocal involvement is highly possible due to the haematogenous route of spread and it may be that the entire spine requires imaging for both forms of osteomyelitis.

Plain radiographs are usually normal within the first 8–10 days. Vertebral end plate involvement is usually subtle and often not detected until disease advancement.

Subtle radiographic features in vertebral osteomyelitis are: disc space narrowing, indistinct end plate changes and possibly periosteal reaction. Later as healing occurs, there may be disk space narrowing or fusion and vertebral body height loss. This can lead to spinal deformity, spinal instability and potential neural compromise. In tuberculous osteomyelitis, the deformity is classically described as a gibbus deformity.

CT imaging has a role and demonstrates bony destruction and involvement of the paravertebral soft tissues and discs.

MR usually has characteristic features and is the imaging modality of choice.

In pyogenic spondylitis/discitis there is a pattern of disc involvement with peridiscal bone destruction and diffuse homogeneous vertebral body enhancement.

The MR features in pyogenic osteomyelitis are:

- T1-weighted images show loss of disc height, low signal in the vertebral bodies due to marrow oedema.
- T2-weighted images demonstrate high signal in the affected disc space and vertebral bodies. The nuclear cleft, normally seen as a linear band of low signal within the intervertebral disc is often effaced. The discs and involved vertebral body will enhance post intravenous contrast. Contrast enhancement may also describe an abscess or phlegmon.

Not surprisingly, the tuberculous spondylodiscitis pattern on MRI reflects the patho-physiological process described earlier. The signal on T1- and T2-weighting will be the same as for pyogenic disease but the distribution pattern will be different.

There is bone destruction with local heterogeneous vertebral body enhancement predominating and relative disc preservation or normal appearance of the disc signal.

Associated paraspinal abscesses are found more commonly in TB, whereas disc abscesses are associated with pyogenic infections.

References

Chang M-C, Wu HTH, Lee C-H et al. Tuberculous spondylitis and pyogenic spondylitis: comparative magnetic resonance imaging features. *Spine* 2006; **31**(7): 782–8.

Cunha BA. Fever of unknown origin: clinical overview of classic and current concepts. *Infect Dis Clin N Am* 2007; **21**: 867–915.

Saifuddin A. *Musculoskeletal MRI*. London: Hodder Arnold; 2008.

Torre JJ, Bohinski RJ, Kuntz C. Vertebral osteomyelitis. *Neurosurg Clin N Am* 2006; **17**: 339–51.

Packet 7 Case 1 Question

KIAT TAN

Clinical history

A 40-year-old male motorcyclist transferred from another hospital after crashing on the motorway. He had undergone a CT scan at the other hospital prior to transfer that, unfortunately, has not been sent with him. You have just performed another CT scan on him. The CT head is normal.

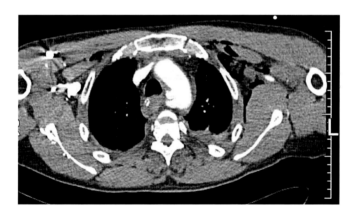

Figure 7.1.1

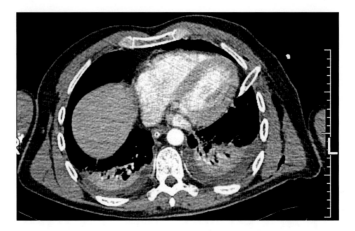

Figure 7.1.2

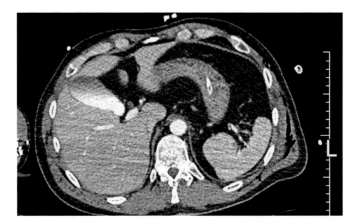

Figure 7.1.3

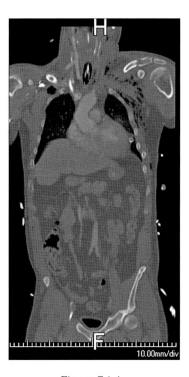

Figure 7.1.4

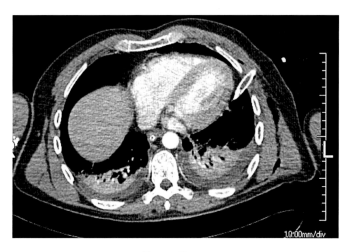

Figure 7.1.5

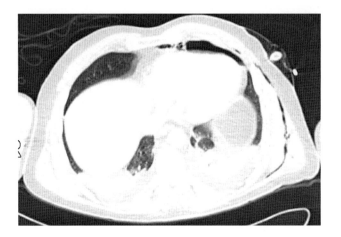

Figure 7.1.6

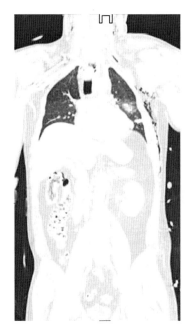

Figure 7.1.7

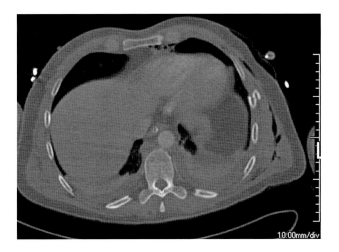

Figure 7.1.8

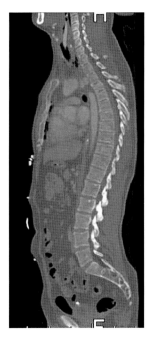

Figure 7.1.9

Packet 7 Case 1 Answer

Model answer

Examination
Selected reconstructed images from a post IV contrast CT chest, abdomen and pelvis.

Findings and interpretations
- Chest drain in situ.
- ET tube in situ.
- NG tube in situ.
- Small left pneumothorax.
- Gas in soft tissue.
- Bilateral pleural effusions.
- Bilateral airspace opacification.
- Thoracic compression fracture (note subtle bulge at T4).
- Left clavicular fracture.
- Left rib fractures.
- Traumatic aortic injury.
- Contrast in gall bladder (presumably from the previous CT scan at another hospital).
- Unusual arterial branch from the right common carotid (seen clearly on the coronal scan).

Diagnosis
Multitrauma with:

(1) Pneumothorax
(2) Traumatic aortic injury
(3) Multiple fractures
(4) Pulmonary contusion
(5) Surgical emphysema
(6) Possible prior poor renal function due to hypoperfusion, as evidenced by contrast in gall bladder.

Management
(1) Needs discussion with cardiologist, cardiothoracic surgeons and interventional radiologist regarding treatment of traumatic aortic injury and the abnormal vascular anatomy.

(2) Inform clinicians of the other injuries.

(3) Consideration for MRI of the spine when more stable in view of the spinal fracture.

(4) Advise clinicians to check fluid balance and renal function (in the unlikely event this has not been done already)

In this case

The patient also has an aberrant right subclavian artery that arises just distal to the site of aortic transaction (not clearly shown). A graft has been inserted into the right common carotid to supply the right upper limb so that the right subclavian can be safely occluded by stenting. Also, the risk of paraplegia is greatly increased if the aorta is clamped proximal to the subclavian (as the subclavian supplies important collaterals to the thoracic cord when the aorta is clamped).

Traumatic aortic injury

This case is similar to the ones with multiple pathologies (including subtle ones) so beloved of FRCR long case examiners.

Traumatic aortic injury (TAI) was first described in 1557 by Vesalius but was relatively uncommon until the advent of motorized transport. Traumatic aortic injury is the second commonest cause of death in road traffic collisions. Other causes of traumatic aortic injury include falls, crush injuries and airplane crashes.

Seventy-five to ninety percent of patients with TAI die at the scene of the collision. Of those who make it alive to hospital, approximately 50% expire prior to definitive treatment. Untreated, only 2–5% of patients survive the acute incident long enough to form aortic pseudoaneurysms. The commonest site of injury is the aortic isthmus (50–80%) although the injury can occur anywhere along the length of the aorta.

The chest radiograph can be useful in the acute setting and in many centres is used for the initial evaluation of mediastinal haematoma or vascular disruption.

The signs to assess for are:

- Widened mediastinum greater than 8 cm ± 25% of the width of the thorax
- Loss of definition of the aortopulmonary window
- Obscuration of the aorta, in particular the transverse aorta
- Rightward deviation of the trachea, oesophagus, NG tube
- Left mainstem bronchus depression
- Left apical cap (blood in the extra-pleural space).

It must be noted that approximately 7% of chest radiographs may be normal and in the clinical setting, further evaluation is warranted.

CT aorta findings include:

- Intimal flap
- Traumatic pseudoaneurysm
- Contained rupture
- Abnormal aortic contour
- Sudden change in aortic calibre (aortic pseudocoarctation)
- Active contrast extravasation (very rare).

CT abdominal findings in the correct clinical settings that may represent thoracic aortic injury include:

- Small calibre aorta
- Retrocrural haematoma.

The patient should then go on to have a CT aorta for further evaluation.

The commonest site of injury is at the aortic isthmus (2 cm from the origin of the left subclavian artery) and seen on the axial CT sequence, along the medial curve of the arch at the level of the left pulmonary artery and left main stem bronchus.

The treatment of choice is between either endovascular stent grafting or open surgical repair. CT imaging with multiplanar reformatting is useful for both surgical and endovascular planning and not just for pure diagnostic work-up. The rationale for endovascular stenting is to prevent further expansion and rupture of the aorta by exclusion of the injury from the high flow rate of the systemic circulation. At present, most centres appear to favour stent grafting, although the long-term follow-up data for this procedure are not yet available. The short-term complications of endovascular stenting include stroke, infection, puncture site pseudoaneurysm, device migration, device collapse and laryngeal nerve damage.

Table of the findings:

Figure 7.1.1: Aortic transection
Figure 7.1.2: Left intercostal drain
Figure 7.1.3: Contrast layering in the gall bladder
Figure 7.1.4: Left clavicular fracture, surgical emphysema left chest wall
Figure 7.1.5: Bilateral pleural effusions
Figure 7.1.6: Pneumothorax and pneumomediastinum
Figure 7.1.7: Pulmonary contusion and left surgical emphysema
Figure 7.1.8: Left rib fracture
Figure 7.1.9: Compression fracture at T4

References

Gleason TG, Bavaria JE. Trauma to the great vessels. In: Cohn LH, ed. *Cardiac surgery in the adult.* New York: McGraw-Hill; 2008: 1333–54.

Samett EJ. Aorta, trauma. Available at: http://www.emedicine.medscape.com/article/416939-overview

Steenburg SD, Ravenel JG, Ikonomidis JS, Schonholz C, Reeves S. Acute traumatic aortic injury: imaging evaluation and management. *Radiology* 2008; **248**: 748–62.

Packet 7 Case 2 Question

INDRAN DAVAGNANAM

Clinical history

A 43-year-old male patient with a known chronic condition presents with worsening balance problems.

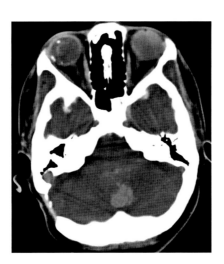

Figure 7.2.1

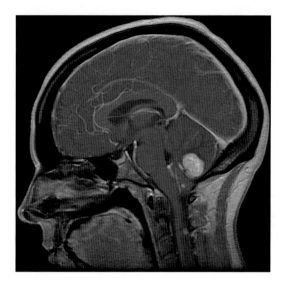

Figure 7.2.2

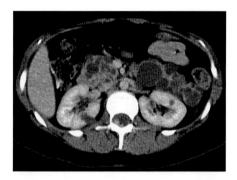

Figure 7.2.3

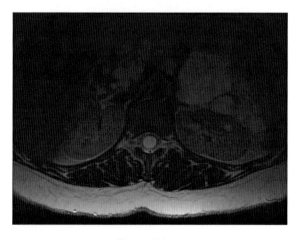

Figure 7.2.4

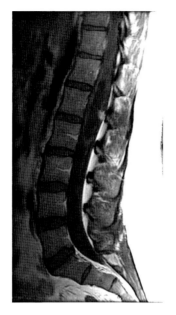

Figure 7.2.5

Packet 7 Case 2 Answer

Model answer

Examinations
- Post-contrast CT brain and abdomen.
- Post-contrast MRI brain and lumbar spine.

Findings
- Post-contrast axial CT image of the brain demonstrates an intra-axial enhancing mass of the left cerebellar hemisphere and vermis. A right posterior fossa craniotomy is noted. There is choroidal/retinal calcification of the right eye. The vitreous of the left globe is hyperdense (Figure 7.2.1).
- Post-contrast sagittal T1-weighted image of the brain demonstrates an enhancing mass involving the inferior vermis of the cerebellum. Further smaller similar lesions are seen in the cerebellar tonsil and upper cervical spinal cord at the level of C2/3 (Figure 7.2.2).
- Post-contrast axial CT of the abdomen showing multiple hypodense cyst-like lesions of the pancreas and other similar hypodense lesions of both kidneys. Right posterior intradural nodular enhancing lesions are seen within the vertebral canal (Figure 7.2.3).
- Axial T2-weighted image at the approximate level of the renal veins demonstrating expansion and central T2-weighted hyperintensity of the spinal cord. The T2-weighted hyperintense cystic lesions of the pancreas and kidneys are noted (Figure 7.2.4).
- Post-contrast sagittal T1-weighted image demonstrating cystic expansion of the terminal spinal cord involving the conus medullaris (T12 to L2) and an enhancing posterior nodule at the level of L1 (Figure 7.2.5).

Interpretations
- Multiple haemangioblastomas; the largest in the cerebellum with smaller haemangioblastomas of cerebellar vermis and cervical spinal cord (C2/3).
- A large cystic haemangioblastoma of the terminal spinal cord.
- Multiple pancreatic and renal cysts.
- Previous right posterior fossa surgery probably for removal of a haemangioblastoma.

- Phthisis bulbi of the right eye probably from recurrent retinal haemorrhage/detachment.
- Possible vitreal/retinal haemorrhage of the left eye.

Diagnosis
Von Hippel-Lindau (VHL) syndrome.

Management
- Urgent ophthalmological referral for management of ocular haemorrhage from retinal angiomas/haemangioblastomas.
- Neurosurgical referral for further neurosurgical management with or without neuro-endovascular embolization.
- MR review of the entire neural axis to document and quantify the number and extent of haemangioblastomas.
- Review of the abdominal viscera in particular the pancreas, kidneys and adrenals for renal cell carcinoma and phaeochromocytomas.
- Imaging follow-up of intra-abdominal and neural axis disease.
- Family screening and counselling.

Von Hippel-Lindau (VHL) syndrome

Von Hippel-Lindau syndrome (VHL) is an autosomal dominant syndrome, which can present with a spectrum of clinical features due to variable expression of the gene. The VHL gene causes inactivation of the tumour suppression gene on chromosome 3 (specifically 3p25.5) resulting in benign and malignant tumours in multiple organs.

VHL manifests with:

- Haemangioblastomas (HBLs); retinal and neural axis
- Cysts of the abdominal viscera (renal, pancreatic, epididymal and endolymphatic sac cysts)
- Pancreatic tumours (serous microcystic adenomas, neuroendocrine tumours and rarely adenocarcinomas)
- Renal cell carcinoma
- Endolymphatic sac tumours
- Epididymal cystadenomas
- Phaeochromocytomas.

Haemangioblastoma (HBL) is a benign vascular tumour according to the classification proposed by Mulliken and Glowacki. It is commonly associated with VHL syndrome but is not a pathognomonic sign. The presence of HBL must be correlated with other major and minor diagnostic criteria for a definite diagnosis of VHL. This has significant implications for both the individual and their family, especially if there is no family history of the disorder. As such, imaging plays an important role in screening, lesion detection, lesion follow-up and surveillance of high-risk asymptomatic individuals.

HBLs are cystic tumours with an enhancing solid mural nodule associated with the pial surface. HBLs can also be solid, haemorrhagic or mixed. These tend to demonstrate periods of increased growth on average every 2 years manifesting usually as an increase in size of the cystic component interspersed with periods of arrested growth. On MR they are low signal on T1-weighted, high on T2-weighted with contrast enhancement. Feeding or draining vessels may be demonstrated in the solid component as serpinginous flow voids best seen on T2-weighted imaging.

The earliest clinical presentation of VHL is usually with visual symptoms due to retinal/vitreal haemorrhage from retinal HBLs which themselves are difficult to visualize on cross-sectional imaging. Retinal HBLs on T1-weighted MRI are higher signal than vitreous. Once they are large enough to be conspicuous on CT or MR, they may have already led to visual loss. Annual screening will require ophthalmoscopy with fluorescein angiography. Radiological input for screening retinal lesions is minimal but orbital MR is useful as retinal HBLs have an increased risk of retinal detachment.

Within the neuroaxis haemangioblastomas are typically seen in the cerebellum, spinal cord and the medulla. Cerebellar HBLs are present in about 50% of patients with VHL and tend to recur post-resection. Spinal cord HBLs in VHL occur at a younger age. Syringomyelia often results from cystic HBLs; the imaging differentiation of cystic HBLs from syrinxes can be difficult.

Endolymphatic sac tumours and bilateral lesions are associated in VHL. They are rare slow-growing tumours which cause local bone destruction and new bone formation. They do not metastasize but are locally aggressive. CT demonstrates geographical bone destruction, with speculated intratumoural bone. MR changes show a heterogeneous signal abnormality with heterogeneous enhancement.

Abdominal visceral cysts are a striking feature of the syndrome; close scrutiny to identify visceral tumours on the background of florid cystic disease is often necessary. However CNS involvement is usually prior to renal disease. Renal disease in VHL patients ranges from renal cysts, hyperplastic cysts to renal carcinoma. The full spectrum can occur in a single kidney. Clear cell renal carcinoma in VHL tends to be multicentric or bilateral as well as partly cystic occurring in 40% of patients, usually presenting in patients in their 50s or younger. Renal cell carcinomas (RCCs) in VHL are either solid hypervascular lesions or complex cystic lesions with mural nodules and thick septations. The use of ultrasound as compared with CT will be dependent on several factors:

- Lesions smaller than 2 cm, ultrasound is more sensitive than CT
- In surveillance, ultrasound is preferred, due to the radiation burden from CT
- CT is more helpful than US if there is marked architectural distortion due to scarring.

Phaeochromocytomas are present in a smaller proportion (10–15%) of patients and form the basis for phenotypic differentiation of the syndrome. Similar to RCCs, VHL-associated phaeochromocytomas present at a younger age, in multiple, bilateral and ectopic locations (organ of Zuckerandl, glomus jugulare, carotid body, periaortic, perisplenic and intrarenal regions). CT can demonstrate phaechromocytomas (enhancing complex cystic or solid mass, can have necrosis, haemorrhage or calcification). MR is the preferred modality if an adrenal phaeochromocytoma is suspected whilst 131 metaiodobenzylguanidine (MIBG) is used if both CT and MRI are negative.

References

Atlas SW. *Magnetic resonance imaging of the brain and spine*, Vol I, 4th edn. Lippincott, Williams & Wilkins; 2008: 300–3.

Barkovich AJ. *Pediatric neuroimaging*, 4th ed. Philadelphia: Lippincott, Williams & Wilkins; 2005: 482–6.

Leung RS, Biswas SV, Duncan M, Rankin S. Imaging features of von Hippel-Lindau disease. *RadioGraphics* 2008; **28**: 65–79.

Osborn AG, Blaser S, Salzman K et al. *Diagnostic imaging: brain*, 1st ed. Amirsys/Elsevier; 2004: 86–9.

Smoker W, Gentry LR, Yee NK, Reede DL, Nerad JA. Vascular lesions of the orbit: more than meets the eye. *RadioGraphics* 2008; **28**: 185–204.

Packet 7 Case 3 Question

KATE TAYLOR-ROBINSON

Clinical history

A 6-hour-old baby boy in neonatal ICU with an imperforate anus. Films are requested to check line positions.

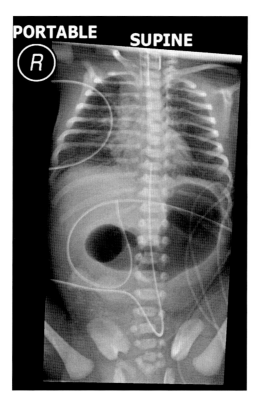

Figure 7.3.1

(a)

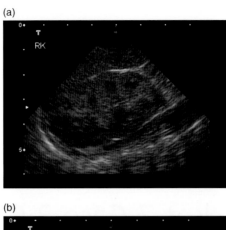

(b)

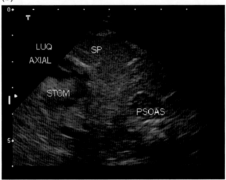

Figure 7.3.2

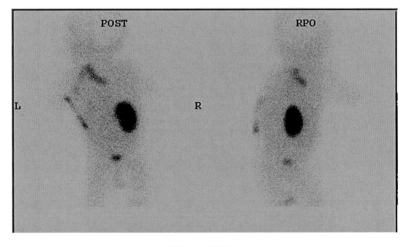

Figure 7.3.3

Answers to follow on page 248

Packet 7 Case 3 Answer

Model answer

Examinations
- Plain radiograph of chest and abdomen (Figure 7.3.1).
- Ultrasound of the right upper quadrant region (Figure 7.3.2a).
- Ultrasound of the left upper quadrant region (Figure 7.3.2b).
- DMSA renogram (Figure 7.3.3).

Findings and interpretations

Plain radiograph
- ET tube in situ – tip at the level of T1 in a satisfactory position.
- Tip of a presumed nasogastric tube captured at the top of the film, which has not been advanced beyond the level of the cervical oesophagus. This suggests obstruction and in a neonate may indicate oesophageal atresia.
- Umbilical artery catheter in situ – tip at the level of T8 in a satisfactory position.
- Umbilical vein catheter in situ – the tip at T10/11 overlying the liver. This should be removed and re-sited, if possible, so that it lies with its tip at the level of the diaphragm.
- The stomach and duodenum are dilated and gas filled with an absence of gas distally. This is the 'double bubble' appearance of duodenal obstruction. In the neonate this may be due to duodenal atresia or stenosis, malrotation or an annular pancreas. The presence of gas within the stomach in the presence of oesophageal atresia would indicate the presence of a tracheo-oesophageal fistula communicating with the part of the oesophagus below the atresia.
- Vertebral segmentation anomalies noted within the sacrum.
- Salient normal findings include twelve normal rib pairs, levocardia and situs solitus.

Ultrasound + DMSA
A normal right kidney is demonstrated on both studies but no left kidney or left kidney function is shown on these images. No large cystic structure is demonstrated in the left upper quadrant (making an obstructed non-functioning kidney unlikely). This is consistent with left-sided renal agenesis.

Diagnosis

Multiple congenital anomalies, likely to represent part of the VATER or VACTERL spectrum (VATER – vertebral defects, imperforate anus, tracheo-oesophageal fistula, radial and renal dysplasia; VACTERL – vertebral, anorectal, cardiac, tracheo-oesophageal fistula, oesophageal atresia and renal, rib and limb/radial anomalies). In this patient, features include: sacral segmentation anomaly, oesophageal atresia, tracheo-oesophageal fistula, duodenal atresia, renal agenesis and anorectal malformation.

Management

This child needs urgent surgical attention. Surgical intervention may involve duodenal repair and defunctioning colostomy. Repair of oesophageal atresia could be delayed. A percutaneous gastrostomy will be required for enteral feeding with consideration given to possible aspiration.

This child will require post-operative imaging after colostomy formation to assess the level of anorectal malformation and any rectovesical fistula. Likewise contrast studies will be required following repair of the duodenal atresia.

Examine the patient and review any other films for the presence of limb abnormalities. Consider echocardiogram to evaluate for any associated cardiac anomalies.

Ultrasound the lumbosacral spine to assess for occult dysraphism.

Discussion

Ideal position for ET tube = T1–T2.

The umbilical arterial line always dips down towards the pelvis entering one of the internal iliac arteries before heading up into the aorta. The tip should ideally lie between T6 and T9 to avoid thrombosis of major arterial branches. Alternatively a low position can be used ideally at L3–4 just above the aortic bifurcation.

The umbilical venous line goes via the umbilical vein, the left portal vein and the ductus venosus to the IVC. The tip should lie at the level of the diaphragm or T7–T8 to ensure it is not intrahepatic.

VATER/VACTERL

VATER and VACTERL are non-random associated congenital anomalies. They occur in 2–13 per 10 000 births and are more common in infants of diabetic mothers and in infants with trisomy 18 (Edward syndrome). VACTERL is also associated with bronchopulmonary foregut malformations such as pulmonary atresia, congenital lobar emphysema and pulmonary sequestration.

Infants presenting with oesophageal atresia with or without a tracheo-oesophageal fistula have associated anomalies of VATER/VACTERL in 20% of cases. Thus further investigation will most probably be required. Prenatal finding of polyhydramnios and absent stomach 'bubble' with fluid-filled loops of bowel on ultrasound can suggest oesophageal atresia. Post-natally, symptoms, which are suggestive include: excess salivation, regurgitation, choking following attempts at feeding and respiratory distress. Attempts at passing a nasogastric tube will usually be unsuccessful and as such initial assessment with chest, abdomen, pelvis and spine plain films will be essential. The features seen on plain radiograph of oesophageal atresia are an air-filled blind pouch and no distal bowel gas shadowing. If there is an associated distal tracheo-oesphageal fistula, then air in the bowel will be demonstrated and aspiration pneumonia may be seen there also. Further delineation of the subtype of oesophageal atresia can be assessed under fluoroscopic contrast study.

Other associations include congenital scoliosis, which can be demonstrated on plain radiography along with vertebral anomalies.

These congenital features may be picked up in utero, in particular limb anomalies may be unexpectedly detected on prenatal ultrasound by findings of intrauterine growth retardation and short long bones.

In essence, if an unexpected congenital anomaly is found either pre- or post-natally, further features should be sought.

References

Achildi O, Grewal H. Congenital anomalies of the esophagus. *Otolaryngol Clin N Am* 2007; **40**: 219–44.

Durkin EF, Shaaban A. Commonly encountered surgical problems in the fetus and neonate. *Pediatr Clin N Am* 2009; **56**: 647–69.

Grimme JD, Castillo M. Congenital anomalies of the spine. *Neuroim Clin N Am* 2007; **17**: 1–16.

Koifman A, Nevo O, Toi A et al. Diagnostic approach to prenatally diagnosed limb abnormalities. *Ultrasound Clinic* 2008; **3**: 595–608.

Lachman RS. *Taybi and Lachman's radiology of syndromes, metabolic disorders and skeletal dysplasias*, 5th ed. Philadelphia: Mosby Elsevier; 2007.

Slovis TL. *Caffey's pediatric diagnostic imaging*, 11th ed. Philadelphia: Mosby Elsevier; 2008: 1614–7.

Packet 7 Case 4 Question

OLGA HATSIOPOULOU

Clinical history

A 32-year-old woman presents with vague right-sided pelvic pain.

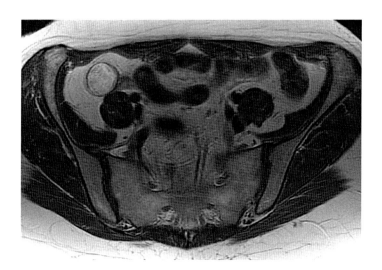

Figure 7.4.1

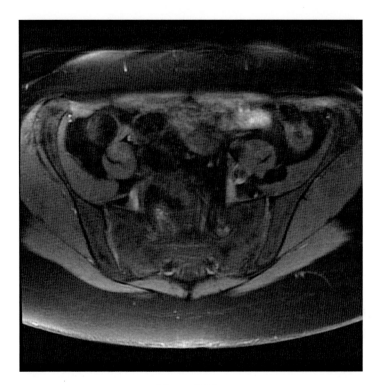

Figure 7.4.2

Answers to follow on page 254

Packet 7 Case 4 Answer

Model answer

Examination
Axial T1-weighted MR pelvis (Figure 7.4.1).
Axial T1-weighted fat saturated MR pelvis (Figure 7.4.2).

Findings and interpretations
- A well-circumscribed 3 × 3.5 cm round mass located in the right adnexum. Just medial and adjacent to this mass, there are several small low T1-weighted signal intensity ovarian follicles.
- The mass is of high signal intensity on the T1-weighted sequence and shows loss of the high signal following fat saturation consistent with the presence of macroscopic fat in the lesion.
- The lesion is unilateral and there is no free fluid in the pelvis.

Diagnosis
- Right ovarian dermoid (mature teratoma).
- The lesion appears non-aggressive and there are no features to suggest complications such as rupture or torsion.

Differential diagnosis
In a patient of this age, differential diagnosis includes endometrioma and haemorrhagic cyst, although these will not result in loss of high signal following fat suppression.

Management
- Referral to the gynaecological team.
- Small (less than 6 cm) uncomplicated dermoids may be managed non-surgically. If symptomatic and growing, surgical excision with ovarian conservation is advocated.

Ovarian dermoid (mature cystic teratoma of the ovary)

Ovarian dermoids are congenital tumours composed of cells from either two or all three germ cell layers. These are benign lesions, the most common ovarian tumour,

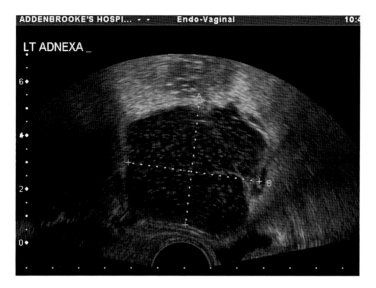

Figure 7.4.3 Endovaginal ultrasound, demonstrates a hypoechoic mass in the left adnexum.

and are most commonly seen during the reproductive years. There is report of up to a 2% risk of malignant degeneration seen in the older age group, in the 6th or 7th decade of life and in larger lesions. Bilateral dermoids are reported in the range of 8–14% and an average size of 5–7 cm and can reach up to 20 cm.

Dermoids are usually asymptomatic but can present with abdominal ± pelvic pain. If the cyst is large or enlarging, patients may present with increasing abdominal girth, pressure symptoms on adjacent structures (constipation, urinary frequency) and uterine bleeding. Patients may present with an acute abdomen if complications occur, such as rupture (chemical peritonitis), infection or torsion.

Dermoids usually contain sebaceous material but can contain any elements arising from all three germ layers including neural tissue, intestinal mucosa and even thyroid tissue.

Imaging investigations will initially depend on the clinical presentation but usually a pelvic ultrasound is the initial imaging investigation of choice especially in a pre-menopausal female. The usefulness of an abdominal radiograph should be borne in mind as the presence of teeth in the lesion provides a high degree of diagnostic confidence.

Ultrasound (US) features depend also on the components of the lesion as well as the size. US may show a completely echogenic mass (Figure 7.4.3) or a cystic lesion with an echogenic shadowing nodule (dermoid plug). The characteristic 'tip of the iceberg' sign describes the echogenic dermoid associated with posterior acoustic shadowing due to the presence of fat and hair components in the lesion. Rupture is suggested by detection of fluid or calcification outside the cyst and if there is peritonitis.

In general worrying features of ovarian masses include solid components, nodules and thick irregular septations, and large size greater than 8 cm will require further investigation in order to exclude the risk of malignancy. Typically endovaginal ultrasound is great for interrogating suspicious features: vascularity within mural nodules, mural irregularities and septations.

CT will show fat attenuation within an ovarian cyst and teeth or calcification. Fat fluid interface can also be seen in lesions on CT.

In uncertain cases small endometriomas can mimic a small dermoid and the converse is true. MRI could assist and Figures 7.4.1 and 7.4.2 demonstrate the characteristic imaging finding of the high T1-weighted signal present in the lesion followed by signal loss with a fat saturation technique corresponding to the fat/sebaceous component. This readily differentiates a dermoid lesion from endometriomas and haemorrhagic cysts. The blood products in these lesions may also be of high signal on T1-weighted sequence (methaemoglobin) but do not suppress following a T1-weighted fat saturation sequence.

As mentioned earlier dermoids may also contain bone, hair or calcifications and these will be of low signal on T1- and T2-weighted sequences.

The fat component can also be of high signal on T2-weighted images.

All imaging may show complications.

Torsion is suggested by the presence of engorged vessels on US and rim enhancement on T1-weighted images. Rupture of a dermoid is confirmed by the presence of high signal T1-weighted fatty sebaceous material within the peritoneal cavity that suppresses on fat suppression sequences.

References

Boyle KJ, Torrealday S. Benign gynaecologic conditions. *Surg Clin of N Am* 2008; **88**: 245–64.

Hricak H, Akin O, Sala E, Levine D. *Diagnostic imaging: gynecology*, 1st ed. Amirsys/Elsevier; 2007: 7–22.

Jain KA. Gynecologic causes of acute pelvic pain: ultrasound imaging. *Ultrasound Clin* 2008; **3**: 1–12.

Park SB, Kim JK, Kim K-R, Cho K-S. Imaging findings of complications and unusual manifestations of ovarian teratomas. *RadioGraphics* 2008; **28**(4): 969–83.

Poder L, Qayyum A, Goldstein RB. Use of MR imaging for further evaluation of sonographically detected adnexal pathology. *Ultrasound Clin* 2006; **1**: 357–83.

Stany MP, Hamilton CA. Benign disorders of the ovary. *Obstet Gynecol Clin N Am* 2008; **35**: 271–84.

Tamai K, Koyama T, Saga T et al. MR features of physiologic and benign conditions of the ovary. *Eur Radiol* 2006; **16**(12): 2700–11.

Packet 7 Case 5 Question

JOHN CURTIS

Clinical history

A 40-year-old female presents with progressive dyspnoea.

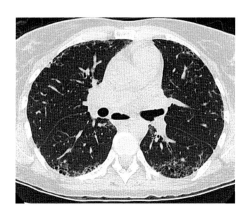

Figure 7.5.1

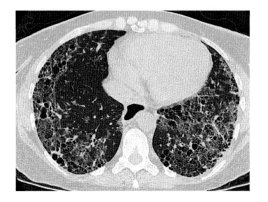

Figure 7.5.2

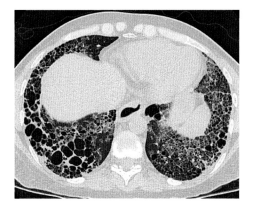

Figure 7.5.3

Answers to follow on page 260

Packet 7 Case 5 Answer

Model answer

Examination
Selected images from an HRCT scan of the chest.

Findings and interpretations
- There is peripheral ground glass change and honeycombing of both lung bases, most marked at the bases.
- There is oesophageal dilatation.

Diagnosis
Scleroderma lung.

Management
- The results are to be communicated to the referring clinican.
- The patient will require referral to the respiratory and rheumatological units if this is the initial presentation.
- Respiratory function testing prior to assessment for possible open lung biopsy.

Progressive systemic sclerosis (scleroderma)

Progressive systemic sclerosis (PSS) is a multisystem connective tissue disorder and like the majority of autoimmune disorders usually affects females. The average age of onset is between 30 and 50 years of age. The disease is characterized by fibrosis, affecting the vascular system in skin, joints, lungs, kidneys, cardiac and the gastro-intestinal tract.

Approximately two-thirds of patients will have pulmonary symptoms. Fibrosis may be suggested in late/advanced disease on plain radiograph with interstitial shadowing affecting the bases and volume reduction. However, HRCT is the imaging modality of choice and ground glass shadowing, septal thickening and vague sub-pleural nodules are early features. Previous imaging is very useful in assessing the progression of fibrosis which, in the case of scleroderma, is usually slower than that seen in usual interstitial fibrosis (UIP). The radiological appearances may otherwise be indistinguishable, although UIP is more likely than scleroderma to be associated with

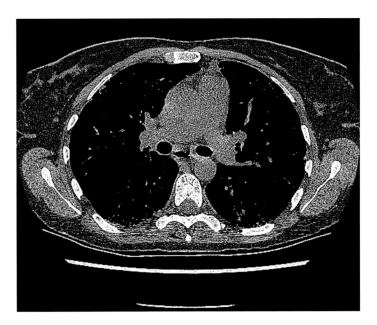

Figure 7.5.4

a coarser pattern of fibrosis and honeycombing. Traction bronchiectasis may result from fibrosis. Scleroderma is associated with mediastinal lymphadenopathy which may progress to egg-shell calcification. Aspiration may result from oesophageal dysmotility and there is a higher incidence of lung cancer in patients with scleroderma-associated fibrosis.

Oesophageal involvement is seen in PSS (50–90%) and a variant of, CREST syndrome. The oesophagus becomes dilatated due to smooth muscle atrophy and sphincter dysfunction. The sphincter dysfunction will also lead to gastro-oesphageal reflux and its complications, both short and long term: oesphagitis, ulcers, strictures and Barrett's disease.

CREST syndrome is so-called because of the presence of calcinosis, Raynaud's phenomenon, oesophageal dysmotility, sclerodactyly and telangiectasia. Dilatation of the oesophagus is not seen in UIP.

Scleroderma may cause pulmonary artery hypertension either as an isolated finding or because of pulmonary fibrosis. This may be suggested by dilatation of the pulmonary trunk (Figure 7.5.4). Older patients with scleroderma (older than 60 years of age) have been found to be at risk for developing pulmonary arterial hypertension. The reason is unknown.

Checklist
When confronted with a chest radiograph or high resolution CT of the chest in patients with basal fibrosis there is a useful checklist which comprises the main causes, all of which are directly or indirectly associated with the letter 'A':

- A – **Alveolitis** of uncertain aetiology (UIP, NSIP).
- A – **Autoimmune**, i.e. rheumatoid lung (look at shoulders for erosions), systemic lupus erythematosus (look for pleuro-pericardial fluid), scleroderma (look at oesophagus and slow progression over time).
- A – **Amiodarone**. This should act as an *aide memoire* to include all drugs implicated in basal fibrosis such as bleomycin, methotrexate, etc. Amiodarone is metabolized in the liver and its iodine content contributes to a dense liver on CT, so look for it.

- **A – Asbestosis**. This is classically a basal pulmonary fibrosis associated with pleural plaques and a positive history of appropriate exposure to asbestos fibres. The fibrosis typically does not progress as quickly as UIP.
- **A – Aspiration**. This tends to be coarse, unilateral or asymmetrical and there may be an associated hiatus hernia.

References

Babyn P, Doria AS. Radiologic investigation of rheumatic disease. *Rheum Dis Clin N Am* 2007; **33**: 403–40.

Mayberry JP, Primack SL, Müller NL. Thoracic manifestations of systemic autoimmune diseases: radiographic and high-resolution CT findings. *RadioGraphics* 2000; **20**: 1623–35.

McArdle JR, Trow TK, Lerz K. Pulmonary hypertension in older adults. *Clin Chest Med* 2007; **28**: 717–33.

Schneider A, Merikhi A, Frank B. Autoimmune disorders: gastrointestinal manifestations and endoscopic findings. *Gastrointest Endoscopy Clin N Am* 2006; **16**: 133–51.

Packet 7 Case 6 Question

JOHN CURTIS

Clinical history

A 49-year-old male presents with haematuria and loin pain.

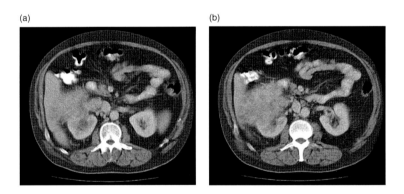

Figure 7.6.1

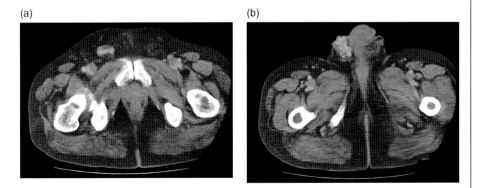

Figure 7.6.2

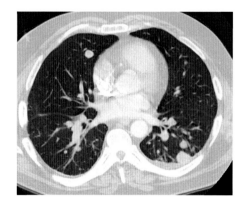

Figure 7.6.3

Ant   Post

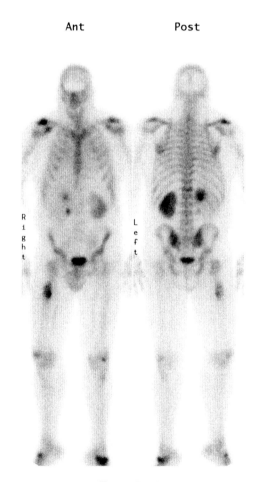

Figure 7.6.4

Answers to follow on page 266

Packet 7 Case 6 Answer

Model answer

Examination
- Selected images from a CT scan of the chest and abdomen post IV and oral contrast.
- Radio-isotope bone scan.

Findings and interpretations
- Exophytic mass lesion right kidney with tumour invasion of the renal vein and inferior vena cava (IVC).
- Enhancing vessels in the right groin in keeping with a varicocele.
- Multiple pulmonary metastases.
- Focal increased tracer uptake proximal right femur.
- Increased uptake left mid foot.
- Increased uptake right shoulder region.
- Reduced uptake lower pole right kidney due to the renal tumour.

Diagnosis
Right renal tumour (most likely renal cell carcinoma) with renal vein and IVC tumour invasion, pulmonary metastases and a probable right femoral metastasis.

Right-sided varicocele.

Management
(1) Right proximal femur radiograph.
(2) Ultrasound scrotum

Renal cell carcinoma

This case demonstrates a plethora of radiological signs that produce a unifying diagnosis. In this case a femoral radiograph demonstrated a destructive lytic lesion in the proximal femur (Figure 7.6.5). This was treated with embolization (Figure 7.6.6) prior to prophylactic orthopaedic pinning.

Up to 40% of renal cell carcinomas (hypernephromas) may be found on routine CT and US and it is vital to search for this lesion during all CT examinations. These incidental renal cell carcinomas tend to be smaller than when asymptomatic

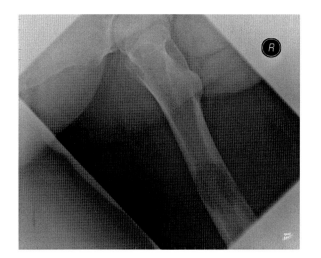

Figure 7.6.5

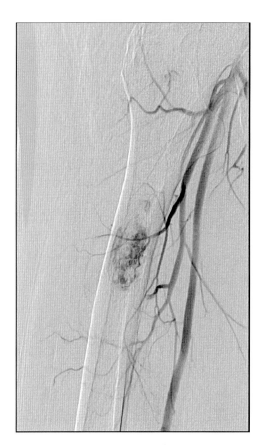

Figure 7.6.6

compared with lesions that cause symptoms. There is a male predominance and there are risk factors which have been found to be associated with developing renal cell carcinoma: smoking, obesity and hypertension. Clinical presentation includes haematuria and flank pain, occasionally with a mass lesion on palpation.

Most renal cell carcinomas are hypervascular on CT imaging and can be calcified in approximately 10% of cases. Right-sided neoplasms may result in varicocele formation in males if the venous return via the right testicular vein is obstructed. The presence of a right-sided varicocele should always raise the suspicion of a right renal mass lesion. This relates to the anatomical difference between the origins of the left and right renal veins. Involvement of the IVC occurs in up to 10% of cases and may even extend into the right atrium in 1%. Right-sided renal tumours are more likely to be implicated in IVC tumour invasion because of the shorter renal vein on that side. Renal vein involvement occurs in up to 35% of cases. Surprisingly, venous involvement does not affect prognosis as long as it can be surgically removed. IVC invasion will usually require further imaging (MRI depending on local availability and expertise) to assess for the extent of tumour extension and pre-operative planning especially in cases with tumour at the level at or above the diaphragm.

Metastases may occur in loco-regional lymph nodes and in the bony skeleton where they are typically lytic and expansile. Lung metastases tend to be of the cannon ball variety. Metastases may also occur in the adrenal glands, muscles and pancreas.

Lytic bone metastases in weight-bearing bones may be treated with embolization prior to prophylactic orthopaedic nailing.

Inspection of the bone scan should include a careful search for absent or partial absence of kidneys which in this case confirms a right renal mass. Diaphyseal increased tracer activity is usually a sign of infiltration in the absence of trauma. Depression of the right kidney may be an indirect marker for hepatomegaly.

References

DeCastro GJ, McKiernan JM. Epidemiology, clinical staging, and presentation of renal cell carcinoma. *Urol Clin N Am* 2008; **35**: 581–92.

Federle MP. *Diagnostic imaging: abdomen*. Amirsys/Elsevier; 2004.

Ng CS, Wood CG, Silverman PM et al. Renal cell carcinoma: diagnosis, staging, and surveillance. *AJR* 2008; **191**: 1220–32.

Wotkowicz C, Wszolek MF, Libertino JA. Resection of renal tumors invading the vena cava. *Urol Clin N Am* 2008; **35**: 657–71.

Packet 8 Case 1 Question

KIAT TAN

Clinical history

A middle-aged gentleman presents with sudden onset chest pain. Aortic dissection?

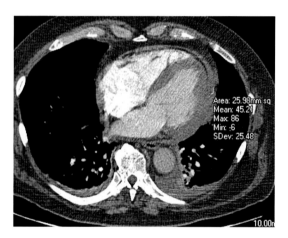

Figure 8.1.1

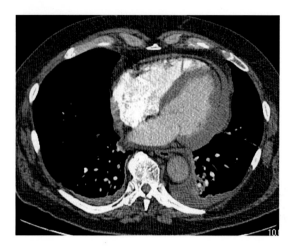

Figure 8.1.2

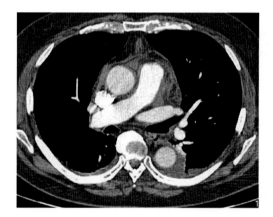

Figure 8.1.3

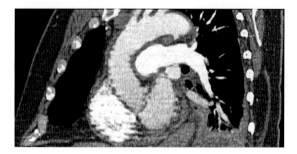

Figure 8.1.4

Answers to follow on page 272

Packet 8 Case 1 Answer

Model answer

Examination
Selected reconstructed images from a post-contrast chest CT.

Findings and interpretations
- High attenuation fluid in the pericardial space.
- The aorta is thick walled.
- Irregular out-pouching on the inferior surface of the aortic arch.
- Bilateral pleural effusions, larger on the left.

Diagnosis
Type A acute intramural haematoma due to a penetrating aortic ulcer.

Differential diagnosis
Type A acute intramural haematoma with a ductus diverticulum.

Management
(1) Urgent referral to the cardiologists/cardiothoracic surgeons.
(2) Urgent echocardiogram as a pre-operative baseline measurement, to rule out tamponade and to assess aortic valve function.

Discussion
The presence of an outpouching on the undersurface of the aortic arch could be a normal variant due to a ductus diverticulum. However, the presence of surface irregularity within the lesion and intramural haematoma makes it unlikely to be a ductus diverticulum.

Acute aortic syndromes

Acute intramural haematoma is part of the spectrum of conditions that form the 'acute aortic syndromes'. These related conditions include penetrating aortic ulcer, acute intramural haematoma, aortic aneurysmal leak/rupture, traumatic aortic injury and aortic dissection. Acute intramural haematoma is classified as either Type A or B according to whether it involves the ascending aorta or not. Type A is treated surgically while Type B can be managed medically. The condition is believed to have a better prognosis than classical aortic dissection. A third of untreated acute ascending aortic haematomas rupture, another third develop into classical dissection and another third 'stabilize'. It should be remembered that up to 55% of the patients who 'stabilize' after the acute episode of intramural haematoma (both Types A and B) subsequently developed aortic aneurysms.

Type B dissection should be treated surgically if there is evidence of progressive aneurysmal dilatation of the aorta. Some surgeons also advocate surgical repair if there is progressive increase in the size of the haematoma.

The presence of haemopericardium in this case suggests that blood has tracked intramurally across the aortic valve annulus. This may lead to either aortic valve incompetence or cardiac tamponade.

Acute intramural haematoma can be reliably distinguished from mural thrombus and aortic dissection by the use of a three-phase CT study. Intramural haematoma tends to lie subintimally **superficial** to any calcification while mural thrombus is **deep** to intimal calcification. A non-contrast-enhanced scan would distinguish between radiodense blood and the more radiolucent thrombus. The arterial and delayed phases can easily help distinguish between the aortic intramural haematoma and dissection.

References
Reece TB, Green GR, Kron IL. Aortic dissection. In: Cohn LH, ed. *Cardiac surgery in the adult*. New York: McGraw-Hill; 2008: 1195–222.

Salvolini L, Renda P, Fiore D et al. Acute aortic syndromes: role of multidetector row CT. *Eur J Radiol* 2008; **65**: 350–8.

Packet 8 Case 2 Question

INDRAN DAVAGNANAM

Clinical history

A 3-year-old presents with recurrent episodic seizures.

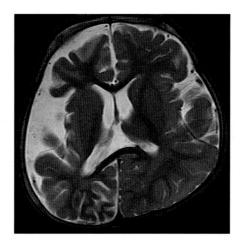

Figure 8.2.1

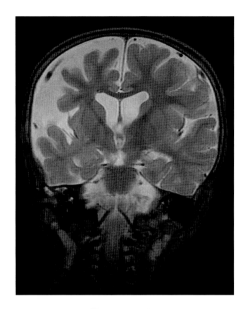

Figure 8.2.2

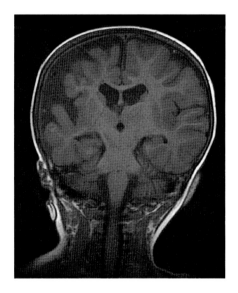

Figure 8.2.3

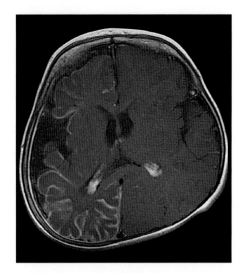

Figure 8.2.4

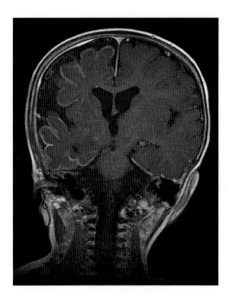

Figure 8.2.5

Answers to follow on page 278

Packet 8 Case 2 Answer

Model answer

Examination
Pre- and post-contrast MRI brain.

Findings
- Pre-contrast axial T2-weighted, coronal T2-weighted and T1-weighted images demonstrating right cerebral hemispheric volume loss compared to the left (Figures 8.2.1 to 8.2.3). The overlying calvarium is slightly thicker than the left. Asymmetry of the head is noted. No asymmetry of myelination is seen.
- Post-contrast axial and coronal T1-weighted images showing leptomeningeal gyriform enhancement of the whole right visualized cerebral hemisphere (Figures 8.2.4 and 8.2.5). No asymmetry or prominence of the choroid plexus is identified.

Interpretations
- Extensive right cerebral hemispheric pial angioma.
- Right cerebral hemispheric volume loss and skull vault thickening.
- Plagiocephaly.

Diagnosis
Right cerebral hemispheric Sturge-Weber syndrome with chronic involutional change of the affected hemisphere.

Management
Review of the intracranial MR imaging assessing extent of pial angiomatous involvement on the ipsilateral side and contralateral involvement if any as well as for ocular choroidal angiomata.

Sturge-Weber syndrome

Sturge-Weber syndrome (SWS) is a sporadic congenital neurocutaneous syndrome with variability in the clinical expression. Both sexes are equally affected. It has a spectrum of clinical and radiological expression. Seizures, hemiparesis, hemianopia, glaucoma and mental retardation constitute the clinical syndrome with normal mental development until the onset of seizures.

SWS is also known as encephalotrigeminal angiomatosis or meningiofacial angiomatosis. Its features consist of facial angiomatosis (or port wine stain), angiomatosis of the eye choroid and leptomeninges. The brain is primarily affected by pial angiomatosis which comprises small venous channels confined to the pia mater and/or meningeal tangle of multiple capillaries. Contrast-enhanced MRI is most accurate in assessing the extent of the pial angioma (pial enhancement) and is essential in radiological diagnosis of SWS. It is said to characteristically involve the occipital and posterior parietal cortex on the same side as the port wine stain. Pial enhancement in the posterior fossa is an atypical finding but is described and does not detract from the diagnosis.

Alongside pial angiomas, there is lack of the superficial cortical venous system, which contributes to venous hypertension and disturbance in normal haemodynamics of the brain. This results in subsequent sequelae: ischaemia, infarction, venous occlusion/thrombosis and atrophy. The affected cerebral hemisphere(s) eventually becomes atrophic in most patients with cranial asymmetry often resulting from cerebral hemiatrophy. In the majority of cases, the cranial vault will demonstrate hemiatrophy; however an enlarged hemicranium can be seen, due to paradoxical increase from underlying subdural collections.

The leptomeningeal malformation is usually on the same side as the port wine stain. There is no correlation in the size of the port wine stain and the underlying brain abnormalities. The presence of a port wine stain in the distribution of the ophthalmic division of the trigeminal nerve should alert the clinician for further investigation. The maxillary and mandibular divisions are less commonly involved. Children with port wine stains involving V_1 may have increased risk of ophthalmic complications.

Cortical calcifications are chronic sequelae, located subjacent to the angioma. They have a gyriform appearance, and are classically described as 'tram track calcifications'. They were described as such when the era of skull radiography was more prevalent but are readily demonstrated on CT. The pathophysiology of cortical calcification has not been established but is thought to be probably due to chronic ischaemia from impaired venous drainage. The calcification is seen frequently posteriorly in the temporo-parietal-occipital areas and is the most frequent finding on CT. Calcification may mask the degree of pial enhancement on CT; in which case, further assessment with MR is necessary.

The choroid plexus is frequently enlarged due to hyperplasia and is seen as a prominent enhancing choroid ipsilateral to the angioma. They can also be calcified and thus may not demonstrate any enhancement.

Angiomas of the choroid and sclera are seen in about 30% of Sturge-Weber syndrome patients. Due to immaturity, the globe responds to increased intraocular pressure with an enlarged globe (buphthalmos) which in some children is present at birth. The presence of choroidal angioma correlates with the presence of bilateral disease and with the extent of facial involvement.

Angiomas of extremities and viscera are uncommon and represent either an overlap or an extension of Sturge-Weber syndrome known as Klippel-Trenaunay-Weber syndrome.

Quantifying the extent of the intracranial angioma is critical in determining the patient's prognosis; therefore contrast-enhanced MRI should be performed in all patients for whom surgery for seizure control is planned. Prognosis is poor when both of the cerebral hemispheres or the majority of a single hemisphere is involved.

References

Adams ME, Aylett SE, Squier W, Chong W. A spectrum of unusual neuroimaging findings in patients with suspected Sturge-Weber Syndrome. *AJNR* 2009; **30**: 276–81.

Atlas SW. *Magnetic resonance imaging of the brain and spine*. Lippincott, Williams & Wilkins. Volume I;II: 398–402.

Barkovich AJ. *Pediatric neuroimaging*, 4th ed. Philadelphia: Lippincott, Williams & Wilkins; 2005: 476–81.

Chen H. *Atlas of genetic diagnosis and counselling*. Totowa, NJ: Humana Press; 2006: 939–41.

Osborn AG, Blaser S, Salzman K et al. *Diagnostic imaging: brain*, 1st ed. Amirsys/Elsevier; 2004 I;1: 94–7.

Smirniotopoulous JG. Neuroimaging of phakomatoses: Sturge-Weber syndrome, tuberous sclerosis, von Hippel-Lindau syndrome. *Neuroimag Clin N Am* 2004; **14**: 171–83.

Packet 8 Case 3 Question

ALICE POCKLINGTON

Clinical history

A 54-year-old woman is referred to a 'One-Stop' clinic with a right breast lump.

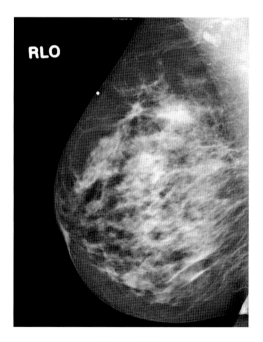

Figure 8.3.1

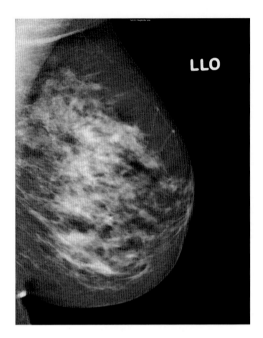

Figure 8.3.2

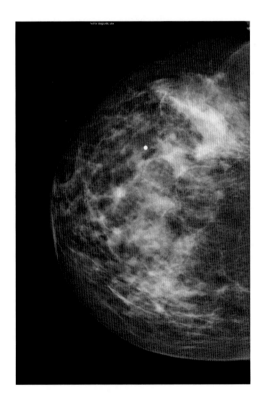

Figure 8.3.3

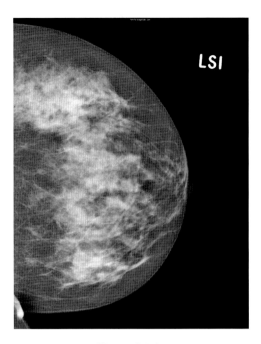

Figure 8.3.4

Packet 8 Case 3 Answer

Model answer

Examination
Standard bilateral two-view mammograms.

Findings and interpretations
- The breasts are of predominantly glandular density bilaterally.
- A radio-opaque marker in the upper outer quadrant of the right breast indicates the site of recent fine needle aspiration (FNA).
- In the upper outer quadrant of the right breast there is a partially spiculate opacity measuring approximately 3 mm in maximum diameter.
- The appearance is suspicious for a carcinoma.
- There are no other suspicious features bilaterally, but the breasts are dense.

Diagnosis
Right breast – M4, suspicious, probably malignant.
Left breast – M2, normal (within the limits of dense breasts).

Differential diagnosis
A radial scar may have a similar appearance, but the management will be the same.

Management
This patient will require triple assessment. If the results of the FNA are equivocal (C4 or less), core biopsy is required.

As the breasts are of glandular density, further similar lesions of a multifocal carcinoma cannot be excluded. Magnetic resonance imaging of both breasts is recommended.

In the case above
The patient had an MRI scan of both breasts, which showed an area of abnormality in the right breast, corresponding to the area of mammographic abnormality, but measuring 37.7 mm (Figure 8.3.5). The lesion demonstrated a malignant enhancement curve (Figures 8.3.6a and b). No other lesions were demonstrated.

The patient had a wide local excision. Pathologically, the lesion was a grade 3 invasive ductal carcinoma, associated with high-grade ductal carcinoma in situ.

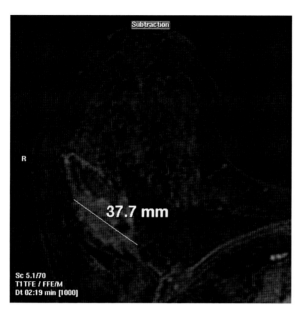

Figure 8.3.5 MRI of the right breast demonstrates an area of abnormality in the outer breast measuring 37.7 mm in maximum diameter.

(a) (b)

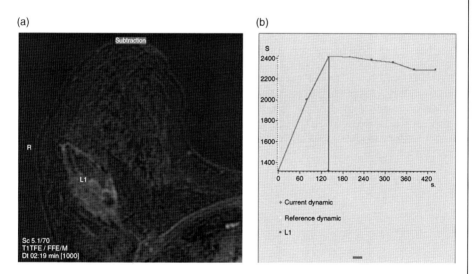

Figure 8.3.6 (a) The region of interest used for plotting the enhancement curves. (b) A malignant-type curve, with a rapid rise in post-gadolinium enhancement, with a subsequent washout phase.

Breast carcinoma and magnetic resonance imaging

Magnetic resonance imaging (MRI) of the breast was first performed in the 1980s, on women with proven breast carcinoma. At the time it was difficult to determine the difference between benign and malignant contrast enhancement.

With the development of faster imaging techniques, it was demonstrated that malignant lesions enhance rapidly, doubling the signal intensity in the first 2 minutes post-contrast (Figure 8.3.6b). Most benign lesions enhance gradually, except fibroadenomata. A fibroadenoma will also enhance rapidly, but not as fast as a malignancy.

The second phase of the enhancement curve is also important. A type I curve is typical of a benign lesion, with a gradual, steady rise in signal intensity. A type II curve has an initial sharp rise in signal intensity, followed by a plateau phase. This is suggestive of malignancy. A type III curve has a washout phase, with a drop in signal intensity, after the rapid rise (Figure 8.3.6b). This is typical of a malignant lesion.

The morphology of the lesion is also important. A fibroadenoma has a well-defined, lobulated border with non-enhancing septations. A malignancy is typically irregular with rim enhancement.

Dynamic breast MRI is useful in the further assessment of patients, who at the end of triple assessment, still fall into the equivocal categories 3 and 4 (suspicious, probably benign and suspicious, probably malignant). It is also useful in detecting multifocal and multicentric disease, and the assessment of the contra-lateral breast in mammographically occult disease.

Dynamic breast MRI also has a role in the surveillance of women with a high risk of familial breast cancer. Less than 1% of women fall into this high-risk group, but algorithms are used to calculate the patient's 10-year risk. The calculation is based on the woman's age and her family history of breast cancer. National Institute of Clinical Excellence (NICE) guidelines recommend annual MRI surveillance for the most high-risk patients. Annual breast MRI is also recommended for women who are known to be carriers of the BRCA1 and BRCA2 mutations aged 30–49 years, and carriers of the TP53 mutation aged 20 years and over. Once these women reach the age of 50 years, they return to the NHS Breast Screening Programme (NHSBSP).

References

Fischer U (ed). Indications for MR mammography. In: *Practical MR mammography*. Thieme; 2004: 140–61.

Lee JYM, Morris EA. Breast MRI: a historical overview. In: Morris EA, Liberman L, eds. *Breast MRI diagnosis and intervention*. USA: Springer; 2005: 3–7.

National Institute for Clinical Excellence. Familial breast cancer: the classification and care of women at risk of familial breast cancer in primary, secondary and tertiary care (update). Clinical Guideline 41. London: National Collaborating Centre for Primary Care.

Packet 8 Case 4 Question

MONICA KHANNA

Clinical history

A 22-year-old man presents with back pain which wakes him at night and is relieved by non-steroidal anti-inflammatory medication.

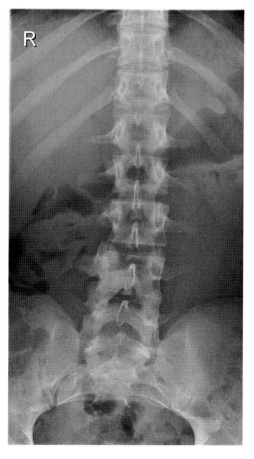

Figure 8.4.1

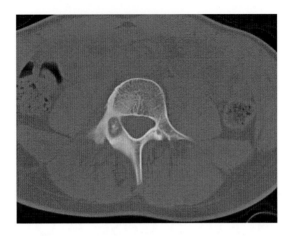

Figure 8.4.2

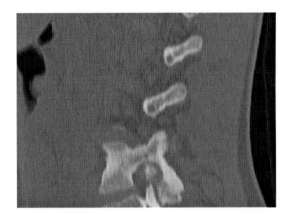

Figure 8.4.3

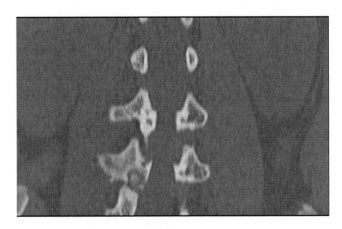

Figure 8.4.4

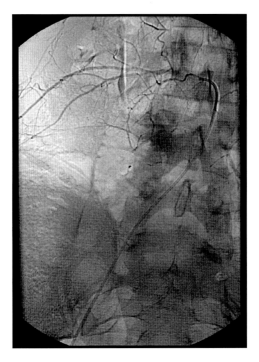

Figure 8.4.5

Packet 8 Case 4 Answer

Model answer

Examinations
- AP lumbar spine radiograph (Figure 8.4.1).
- Axial CT lumbar spine (Figure 8.4.2).
- Sagittal CT lumbar spine (Figure 8.4.3).
- Coronal CT lumbar spine (Figure 8.4.4).
- Angiogram (Figure 8.4.5).

Findings and interpretations

AP lumbar spine
There is an expansile well-circumscribed sclerotic lesion involving the right L4 pedicle, transverse process and right neural arch. There is a mild scoliosis centred at this level, with the lesion at the apex of the concavity.

MDCT lumbar spine
Demonstrates a lesion with a central nidus within the right L4 neural arch with surrounding sclerotic expanded reactive bone extending into the right transverse process and lateral vertebral body. There is matrix mineralization within the lesion.

Angiogram
Demonstrating a blush at the right L4 pedicle.

Diagnosis
Osteoblastoma.

Differential diagnosis
Osteoid osteoma.

Management
Histological confirmation with CT-guided biopsy.
Radical surgical excision is the treatment of choice for osteoblastoma ± pre-operative embolization.

Spinal osteoblastomas

Osteoblastomas are rare, benign bone-forming tumours that are histologically similar to osteoid osteomas, but differ in their size (>1.5–2 cm), are more aggressive and may transform to a malignant entity.

Seventy percent of patients present between the ages of 20 and 30 with a male predominance. They commonly present with localized back pain and may respond to NSAIDs or aspirin. Forty percent occur in the spine, the lumbar spine being most common. Ninety-five percent occur in the posterior elements. Scoliosis associated with osteoblastoma is usually painful and often occurs with the lesion occurring at the apex of the concavity.

Usually congenital scoliosis has a female predominance and is non-painful. These differences should allow differentiation and inform you that the cause should not be attributed to congenital scoliosis.

Radiographically there are three possible patterns which occur in the following descending frequency: lucent expansile lesion (50%), sclerotic lesion (30%) and mixed appearance in the remaining 20%. Twenty-five percent of patients may demonstrate more aggressive features such as cortical thinning, expansion of the bone and the presence of a soft-tissue mass.

MDCT continues to be the investigation of choice for the characterization and local staging of suspected spinal osteoblastomas. Enhanced CT demonstrates typical enhancement of the central vascular nidus.

The MRI appearances of spinal osteoblastomas are varied due to varied content of matrix and osteoid formation and show no characteristic feature. Approximately 50% of osteoblastomas in the spine contain matrix mineralization.

However the role and strength of MRI is in assessment of the adjacent soft tissue. Extensive reactive marrow and soft tissue changes are often seen as high T2 signal, which may overestimate the size of the lesion.

MRI can also demonstrate if there is neural foraminal stenosis and epidural extension from osteoblastomas, and this may explain the higher incidence of neurological dysfunction compared with patients with an osteoid osteoma.

Angiography is not part of the routine set of investigations and the finding of a hypervascular blush is not specific to osteoblastomas.

References

Kan P, Schmidt MH. Osteoid osteoma and osteoblastoma of the spine. *Neurosurgery Clin N Am* 2008; **19**: 65–70.

Shaikh MI, Saifuddin A, Pringle J, Natali C, Sherazi Z. Spinal osteoblastoma: CT and MR imaging with pathological correlation. *Skeletal Radiol* 1999; **28**(1): 33–40.

Wootton-Gorges SL. MRI of primary bone tumors and tumor-like conditions in children. *Radiol Clin N Am* 2009; **47**: 957–75.

Packet 8 Case 5 Question

OLGA HATSIOPOULOU

Clinical history

A 68-year-old female presents with pelvic pain.

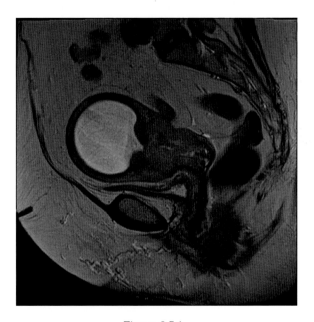

Figure 8.5.1

Answers to follow on page 294

Packet 8 Case 5 Answer

Model answer

Examination
T2-weighted sagittal MR pelvis.

Findings and interpretations
- There is a high signal irregular mass centered in the cervix and extending into the endocervical canal and uterus. The mass is causing obstruction at the endocervical canal and distension of the uterus with fluid (hydrometra).
- The bladder is empty and there is no obvious involvement of the perivesical fat or bladder by the mass.

Diagnosis
Cervical carcinoma.

This is an advanced tumour invading the uterus and is associated with a hydrometra.

Differential diagnosis
Differential diagnosis of a cervical mass includes cervical polyp, although in this case invasion of the uterus by the mass indicates the presence of an aggressive malignant lesion and not a polyp. Other aggressive cervical tumours include cervical lymphoma and metastasis to the cervix.

Management
- Urgent referral to the gynaecological team and assessment via a multidisciplinary approach.
- US of the renal tract to exclude/confirm hydronephrosis.
- MRI for local tumour staging and CT chest and abdomen for distant metastasis detection.
- Local staging is important in treatment decision-making as early confined disease can be treated with radical surgery; advanced disease is treated with chemo radiotherapy.

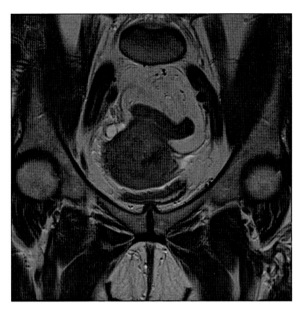

Figure 8.5.2 Coronal pelvic T2-weighted MRI demonstrating irregularity and extension into the right parametrium.

Cervical carcinoma

Cervical carcinoma is the third most common gynaecological malignancy and is the second most common female cancer worldwide. It is associated with low socioeconomic status, human papilloma virus (HPV) and multiple sexual partners. HPV infection in particular is thought to play a major role in the development of cervical carcinoma. It is commonly asymptomatic but may present with abnormal vaginal bleeding or discharge, pelvic pain or urinary symptoms if the bladder is involved or there is pressure effect from a large tumour. Routine screening provides another route of detection, usually detecting pre-malignant dysplasia and allowing diagnosis at an earlier stage. Over recent years there has been the development of several different vaccines, which targets against certain strains of HPV. Hopefully this should help reduce the incidence of cervical carcinoma.

The majority of cervical carcinoma is squamous cell type (85%) with a smaller percentage (15%) consisting of adenocarcinoma, adenosquamous, undifferentiated carcinomas and sarcomas. It is staged clinically using the Federation of Gynecology & Obstetrics (FIGO) staging system. MRI has reasonable accuracy and reasonable correlation with the FIGO staging system of cervical carcinoma and is the imaging of choice for tumour detection and local staging.

The T2-weighted sequence is the most useful sequence (Figure 8.5.2). Cervical tumour is seen as a high signal intensity mass on T2-weighted images. Infiltration of the normally low signal intensity cervical stroma, or invasion of the normally low signal parametrial tissues and vagina can be assessed.

An important point to appreciate is the critical stage for determining if a patient is a suitable surgical candidate; this stage is IIA. If the disease is staged higher than IIA the option is radiotherapy alone. Stage IIA is defined as invasion into the upper two-thirds of the vagina and on MRI this is demonstrated as loss of the normal low signal in the vaginal wall. The next important level of disease stage is stage IIB where involvement of the parametrium is to be ascertained. Greater than or equal to stage IIB, treatment is combined chemotherapy and radiotherapy.

The role of ultrasound in this aspect of gynaecological malignancies is limited. It is not an effective imaging tool due to poor tissue resolution and not effective enough for the assessment of the pelvic side walls.

The role of CT is limited in local disease assessment but has a role in the detection of distant metastases and radiation therapy planning.

References

Akin O, Mironov S, Pandit-Taskar N, Hann LE. Imaging of uterine cancer. *Radiol Clin N Am* 2007; **45**: 167–82.

Brown MAR, de Abreu H. MR imaging of malignant uterine disease. *Magn Reson Imaging Clin N Am* 2007; **14**: 455–69.

Gjelsteen AC, Ching BH, Meyermann MW et al. CT, MRI, PET, PET/CT and ultrasound in the evaluation of obstetric and gynaecologic patients. *Surg Clin N Am* 2008; **88**: 361–90.

Hricak H, Akin O, Sla E, Levine D. *Diagnostic imaging: gynecology*, 1st ed. Amirsys/Elsevier; 2007: 7–14, 3–20, 3–22.

Sala E, Wakely S, Senior E, Lomas D. MRI of malignant neoplasms of the uterine corpus and cervix. *AJR Am J Roentgenol* 2007; **188**(6): 1577–87.

Scheidler J, Heuck AF. Imaging of cancer of the cervix. *Radiolog Clin N Am* 2002; **40**(3): 577–90.

Packet 8 Case 6 Question

KATE TAYLOR-ROBINSON

Clinical history

A 3-month-old boy presents with a history of coliform UTI.

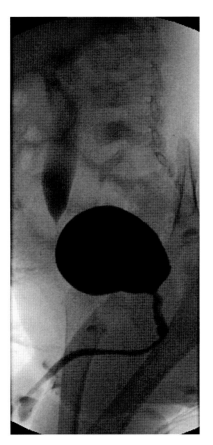

Figure 8.6.1

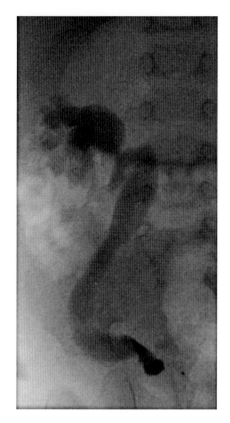

Figure 8.6.2

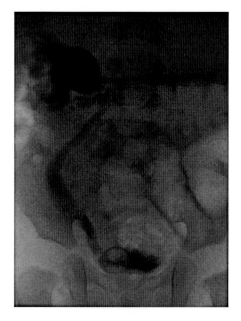

Figure 8.6.3

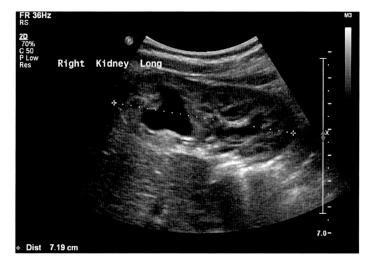

Figure 8.6.4

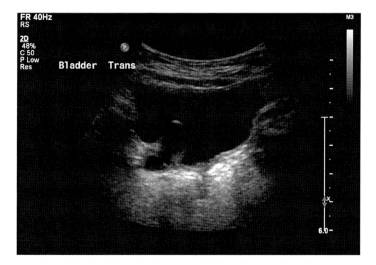

Figure 8.6.5

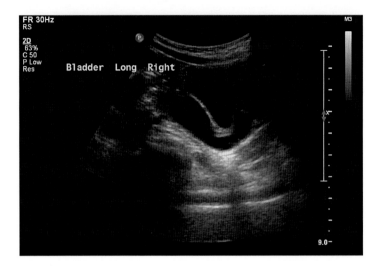

Figure 8.6.6

Answers to follow on page 302

Packet 8 Case 6 Answer

Model answer

Examination
Micturating cystourethrogram (MCUG) and ultrasound of the renal tract:

- Selected images from a micturating cystourethrogram (Figures 8.6.1 to 8.6.3).
- Ultrasound of the right kidney and bladder (Figures 8.6.4 to 8.6.6).

Findings and interpretations

MCUG
- There is right-sided vesicoureteric reflux into a tortuous dilated ureter to the level of the pelvicalyceal system, which is moderately dilated with calyceal blunting (Grade 4 reflux). The pelvicalyceal system has a subtle 'drooping lily' appearance with slight inferior displacement and absence of the upper pole calyces.
- The oblique urethral views during voiding show normal urethra with no evidence of posterior urethral valves.
- The post micturition view shows contrast is still draining from the dilated right system into the bladder and there is a rounded radiolucent filling defect within the bladder.
- This finding indicates reflux into the lower moiety of a duplex right kidney and a coexisting ureterocoele of the distal ureter without reflux.

US
- The right kidney is large for the patient's age and there is hydronephrosis of the upper pole calyces with associated reduction in parenchymal depth.
- A tubular fluid-filled structure is present bulging into the posterior wall of the bladder. This has the appearance of a dilated ureter and ureterocoele.

Diagnosis
Duplex right kidney and ureter with obstructed upper moiety associated with a ureterocoele and reflux into the lower moiety.

Differential diagnosis
There is no differential diagnosis.

Management

Prescribe a treatment course of antibiotics (e.g. trimethoprim) immediately following the MCUG and keep on prophylactic antibiotics thereafter. Refer to a paediatric urologist for further management.

A DMSA scan would be a normal part of the work-up to assess relative renal function and guide management.

Renal duplex

Complete duplex renal anomalies account for 1 in 500 cases. Duplex renal anomalies are associated with Mullerian duct anomalies in the female due to concurrent development and are one of the possible urinary tract abnormalities seen in a female with Mullerian duct anomalies. The renal tract should be evaluated in these cases.

Renal duplex can present through several means pre-natally or post-natally, one of which is a urinary tract infection. In this case, young children with proven urinary tract infections are commonly evaluated with MCUG, US and DMSA. The duplex kidney is larger than a normal kidney with a single collection system and this is seen in this case.

In a renal duplex system, the Weigert-Meyer rule states that the lower moiety ureter inserts in an orthotopic position in the trigone whereas the upper moiety ureter inserts in an ectopic position inferior and medial to this. The upper moiety can insert ectopically in various sites: into the bladder neck, proximal urethra or the vagina. It is prone to ureterocoele formation and obstruction. The lower moiety ureter is prone to reflux due to a shortened tunnel through the bladder wall. If the ureters are dilated, this can be appreciated on ultrasound as well as a ureterocoele which is seen as a circular anechoic structure with a thin echogenic rim. The ureterocoele is demonstrated as a filling defect on the VCUG during the early filling imaging. Other causes of filling defects in the bladder in children are: rhabdomyosarcoma, air bubble, blood clot or fungal ball. However, these would not be associated with a ureterocoele seen at ultrasound or the VCUG.

Subsequent imaging on VCUG can evaluate for the presence of reflux and the presence of a duplex system by abnormal angulation or the ectopic insertion of the ureter.

Management of patients with a duplex system is to minimize long-term renal damage and they will usually require surgical correction of ectopically inserted ureter, especially if there is associated vesico-ureteric reflux.

References
Breech LL, Laufer MR. Mullerian anomalies. *Obstet Gynecol Clin N Am* 2009; **36**: 47–68.
Lane F. *Diagnostic imaging: pediatrics*, 1st ed. /Elsevier Inc. Donnelly; 2005 **5**: 18–21.
Milla SS, Lee EY, Buonomo C, Bramson RT. Ultrasound evaluation of pediatric abdominal masses. *Ultrasound Clin* 2007; **2**: 541–59.

Packet 9 Case 1 Question

KIAT TAN

Clinical history

A baby presents with failure to thrive.

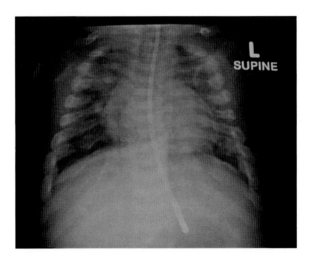

Figure 9.1.1

Answers to follow on page 306

Packet 9 Case 1 Answer

Model answer

Examination
Chest radiograph.

Findings and interpretations
- Multiple rib fractures of varying ages.
- Broad and beaded ribs.
- Lungs clear. No pneumothorax.
- NG tube in situ. Tip of the NG tube is below the diaphragm.

Diagnosis
Severe osteogenesis imperfecta.

Differential diagnosis
Non-accidental injury.

Management
(1) Urgent discussion with paediatricians.
(2) Need to consider skin biopsy + fibroblast culture.
(3) An opinion from an expert paediatric radiologist should be sought.
(4) A skeletal survey is appropriate (but needs specialist input).

Osteogenesis imperfecta

Osteogenesis imperfecta (OI) is a spectrum of genetic disorders due to defects in the production or abnormality of type I collagen resulting in increased bone fragility and defective connective tissues. The altered collagen synthesis leads to joint hypermobility, thin skin, easy bruising and lax joints. The dental structures are also abnormal leading to irregular teeth and discolouration. It is inherited in an autosomal dominant fashion, although most cases are due to spontaneous mutation. The condition is most frequently classified into four clinically distinct subtypes, based on severity and other associated clinical features but it has been further expanded to seven distinct types.

Type	Clinical manifestations
I	Mild disease, short stature, blue sclera
II	Perinatal death
III	Severe disease with deformities: severe scoliosis, triangular face, greyish sclera, abnormal dentition
IV	Moderate disease with deformities: moderate scoliosis, greyish or white sclera, abnormal dentition
V	Moderate disease with deformities: ossification of interosseous membrane of the forearm, radial head dislocation, hyperplastic callus formation

Most patients with OI have a mutation in one or two genes that code for the alpha chains of collagen type 1 (COL1A1 and COL1A2). The diagnosis is usually made by fibroblast culture and analysis of the collagen formed by the cultured fibroblasts. A positive genetic test confirms the diagnosis but the same cannot be said for a negative test. This is due to the possibility that the mutation present was not detected or individuals may have a form of the disorder that is not associated with collagen type 1 mutation and is currently unknown.

The radiological findings include multiple fractures, broad and beaded ribs, broad bones, thinned cortices, thin bones, wormian bones, basilar invagination and cystic metaphysis. Wormian bones are small irregular bones found within the cranial sutures. They are one of the features for OI but not specific as they can occur in other conditions and normality. They are associated with rare conditions: kinky-hair syndrome (Menke's syndrome), acro-osteolysis, cleidocranial dysostosis and Prader-Willi syndrome.

Temporal bone changes also occur, with diffuse resorption of the otic capsule, which has a similar appearance to findings found in otosclerosis.

It must be remembered that non-accidental injury is a more frequent cause of fractures than OI.

The medical management for children with OI is physiotherapy, rehabilitation and orthopaedic surgery. The main function for rehabilitation and physiotherapy is to encourage activity to prevent contractures, disuse atrophy of muscles and immobility-induced bone loss. The fundamental goal of medical management in OI is to reduce fracture rates and prevent long bone deformities with the aim of improving functional outcome. The main pharmacological treatment for OI is bisphosphonate therapy which comprises potent antiresorptive agents and can help relieve chronic bone pain experienced by patients.

References

Ablin DS. Osteogenesis imperfecta: a review. *Can Assoc Radiol J* 1998; **49**: 110–23.

Cremin B, Goodman H, Prax Med M, Spranger J, Beighton P. Wormian bones in osteogenesis imperfecta and other disorders. *Skeletal Radiol* 1982; **8**: 35–8.

Kirpalani A, Babyn PS. *Osteogenesis imperfecta*. Available at: http://www.emedicine.medscape.com/article/411919-overview

Lee DY, Cho TJ, Choi HI et al. Clinical and radiological manifestions of osteogenesis imperfecta type V. *J Korean Med Sci* 2006; **21**: 709–14.

Rauch F, Glorieux FH. Osteogenesis imperfecta. *Lancet* 2004; **363**: 1377–85.

Packet 9 Case 2 Question

ALICE POCKLINGTON

Clinical history

A 52-year-old woman attending NHS breast screening for the first time.

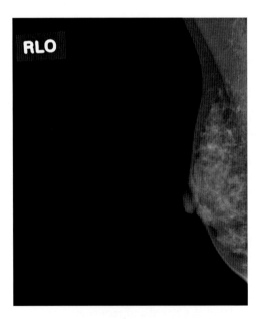

Figure 9.2.1

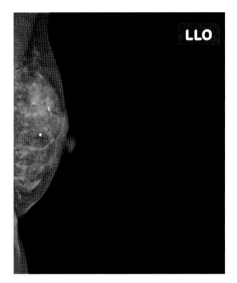

Figure 9.2.2

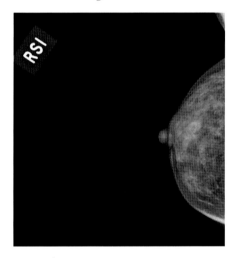

Figure 9.2.3

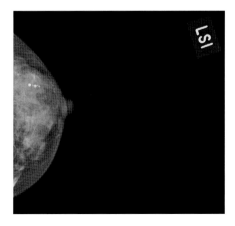

Figure 9.2.4

Packet 9 Case 2 Answer

Model answer

Examination
Standard bilateral two-view mammograms.

Findings and interpretations
- Both breasts are dense and glandular bilaterally.
- A radio-opaque marker indicates the site of the recent fine needle aspiration in the left breast.
- There is extensive micro-calcification in the upper outer quadrant of the left breast. The calcification is variable in size and shape and there are also some linear and branching forms.
- The area of calcification measures 56 mm in maximum diameter. The appearance is of malignant calcification.
- Normal appearance of the right breast.
- Right breast – M1, left breast – M5C (malignant calcification).

Diagnosis
Malignant calcification of the left breast.

Differential diagnosis
There is no differential diagnosis when the calcification is as pleomorphic as in this case.

Management
This patient requires triple assessment, including further views of the left breast. These are lateral mammogram and magnification views of the area of calcification in the cranio-caudal and lateral views.

The left breast should also be examined by ultrasound. If no abnormality is demonstrated on ultrasound, then stereotactic core biopsy of the calcification is necessary.

Referral to the local breast cancer service is required with the results.

In the case above
In this case, further views confirmed the site and malignant appearance of the calcification (see Figures 9.2.5a, b and c).

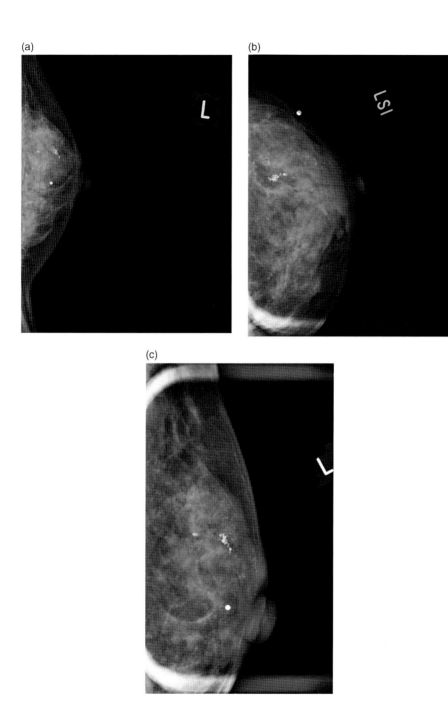

Figure 9.2.5 (a) Lateral mammogram of the left breast. This confirms the localization of the area of abnormality to the upper half of the left breast. (b) Magnified cranio-caudal view of the upper outer quadrant of the left breast. (c) Magnified lateral view of the upper outer quadrant of the left breast. Both of these images confirm the pleomorphic nature of the calcification.

The patient was treated with a mastectomy and axillary node clearance. The pathology was grade 3 invasive ductal carcinoma, with high-grade ductal carcinoma in situ. The total area of abnormality was 58 mm in maximum dimension.

Malignant breast calcification

Half of all mammograms have visible calcifications. Assessment of the morphology and distribution of the calcification is needed in order to determine whether it is benign or malignant.

Magnification views (Figures 9.2.5b and c) are used to assess the morphology of the calcifications. Most calcifications associated with malignancy are less than 0.5 mm in diameter. Malignant calcification is typically either granular or casting. Granular calcification is very small, amorphous and closely grouped together. Clusters of more than five flecks of calcification are suspicious for malignancy. Casting calcifications vary in size and shape and are due to fragments of calcification forming within the ducts. This intraductal formation gives some a typical branching morphology.

A segmental distribution of the calcification is highly suspicious for malignancy, suggesting a single ductal system has been involved. A linear or scattered distribution is less suspicious (Figure 9.2.5c).

One in five breast cancers detected by screening is non-invasive, and the main type of non-invasive breast cancer is ductal carcinoma in situ (DCIS). DCIS is the presence of cytologically malignant epithelial cells within the breast lobular system, with no evidence of invasion. It has a segmental distribution typically and is often multifocal in nature. DCIS may present symptomatically with nipple discharge, or more rarely with a palpable mass, especially in the high nuclear grade category (comedo type). Mammographically, DCIS is calcified in up to 90% of cases, compared to only 30–40% of invasive cancers. This is the fundamental aim of breast screening programmes: to detect non-invasive cancer at an early stage.

Primary treatment of DCIS is surgical excision with clear margins and to remove all foci of suspicious calcification. The recurrence rate is higher in young women, high nuclear grade DCIS and areas of DCIS associated with a palpable abnormality. They are more likely to recur as invasive carcinoma. Mastectomy offers a 98–99% cure for DCIS.

References

Harris JR, Lippman ME, Morrow M, Osborne CK, eds. *Diseases of the breast*, 3rd ed. Baltimore: Lippincott, Williams & Wilkins; 2004: 137.

Menell JH. Ductal carcinoma in situ. In: Morris EA, Liberman L, eds. *Breast MRI, diagnosis and intervention*. Heidelberg: Springer; 2005: 164.

Silva OE, Zurrida S. Benign breast disease. In: *Breast cancer: a practical guide*, 3rd edn. Edinburgh: Elsevier Saunders; 2005: 1–11.

Packet 9 Case 3 Question

JOHN CURTIS

Clinical history

A middle-aged female presents with abdominal pain and swelling.

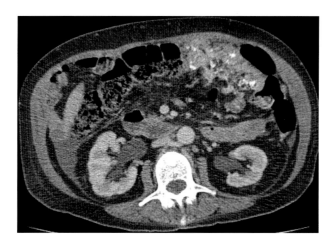

Figure 9.3.1

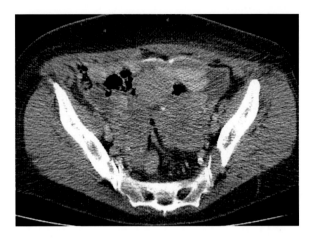

Figure 9.3.2

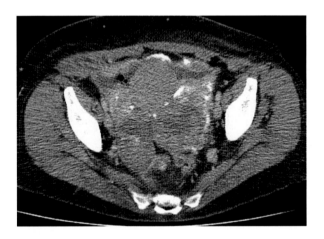

Figure 9.3.3

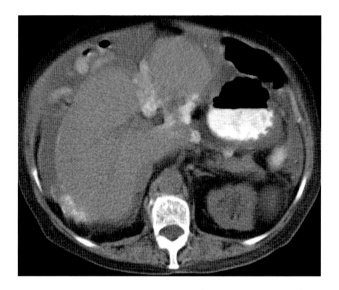

Figure 9.3.4 18 months later.

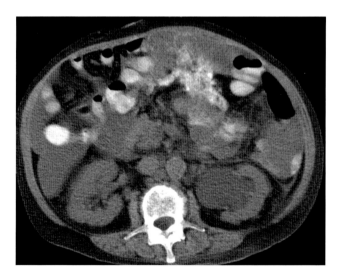

Figure 9.3.5 18 months later.

Packet 9 Case 3 Answer

Model answer

Examination
Selected images from a post-contrast abdominal and pelvic CT with oral contrast.

Findings and interpretations
The initial CT examination demonstrates bilateral ovarian mass lesions (Figure 9.3.2) with peritoneal thickening and calcification (Figure 9.3.3) and omental cake formation (Figure 9.3.1). There is no hydronephrosis.

The scan at 18 months demonstrates left-sided hydronephrosis, calcified omental cake (Figure 9.3.5), and peritoneal calcification over the liver and falciform ligament with ascites. A limited view of the stomach reveals no gross abnormality.

Diagnosis
Omental and peritoneal calcified metastatic disease from bilateral ovarian serous cystadenocarcinomas. Left hydronephrosis indicates distal ureteric encasement on the later study.

Differential diagnosis
Krukenberg ovarian tumours from a primary gastric carcinoma (less likely).

Management
- Ultrasound of left kidney and consideration of a nephrostomy.
- Imaging guided biopsy of omental mass lesion.
- CT chest to assess for distant thoracic metastases.

Ovarian carcinoma

Ovarian carcinoma has a prevalence of up to 50 cases per 100 000 women. It is said that 1 in 70 women will develop a form of ovarian cancer during their lifetime.

Unfortunately none of the available investigations for early ovarian cancer (CA-125, pelvic examination and transvaginal ultrasound) is either sensitive or specific enough to use as a screening tool. At presentation most women are at stage III or stage IV of the disease and will have peritoneal metastases since spread is primarily by direct invasion and peritoneal seeding via peritoneal fluid. Other modes of spread are via the lymphatics causing lymphadenopathy and via the bloodstream.

Fluid circulates through the peritoneal cavity from the pelvis to the diaphragm along peritoneal reflections. There is a propensity for fluid, rich in surface epithelial cells from the ovarian tumour, to accumulate in the subdiaphragmatic regions due to a negative pressure effect caused by respiratory excursions. There are four main areas in the peritoneal cavity where there is a sluggish flow of fluid leading to favoured sites for tumour implantation: the pouch of Douglas, the right lower quadrant, the sigmoid mesocolon and right paracolic gutter (and Morison's pouch). Tumour implants may be very subtle and careful inspection of these areas is essential. They may be solitary or multiple and may coalesce forming 'plaques' that, when large, are termed 'omental cakes'. Enhancement and calcification may occur in these tumour plaques which can lead to diaphragmatic thickening. Liver and splenic involvement tends to cause ill-defined, low density masses which lead to scalloping of these visceral surfaces. The falciform, gastrohepatic and gastrosplenic ligaments may be involved with tumour and may calcify. Bowel and ureteric obstruction are fairly common complications of advanced disease.

Serous cystadenocarcinoma is the commonest histological type and results in peritoneal calcification in a third of cases. The primary ovarian lesion tends to be a multiseptated cyst. Conversely, mucinous tumours tend to be multiloculated and their peritoneal implants do not calcify – in fact they tend to be of low attenuation.

Clinically patients present with pain, bloating and vaginal bleeding. Staging of ovarian cancer is:

I Confined to ovaries
II Extension to pelvic tissues
III Implantation of tumour beyond the pelvis or retroperitoneal lymph node deposits
IV Distant metastases including parenchymal liver deposits

The 5-year survival for stage I disease is 92% and for stage II disease is up to 39%.

Pseudomyxoma peritonei is a histologically benign mucinous tumour that produces thick, viscous mucinous fluid which on imaging resembles ascites except that there is a resulting scalloping of visceral edges. The fluid causes encasement of solid viscera and bowel and carries a very poor prognosis.

Krukenberg tumours are bilateral ovarian metastases and were originally described in patients with a primary mucinous gastric malignancy. Originally thought to occur via transperitoneal spread from only the stomach, it is now thought that any gastrointestinal tumour may give rise to this phenomenon and not exclusively or necessarily via peritoneal spread. Lymphatic and blood-borne spread are thought now to be more likely mechanisms since tumour is found internally within the ovaries and never in the omentum.

References

Harpreet K, Pannu HK, Bristow RE, Montz FJ, Fishman EK. Multidetector CT of peritoneal carcinomatosis from ovarian cancer. *RadioGraphics* 2003; **23**: 687–701.
Woodward PJ, Hosseinzadeh K, Saenger JS. From the Archives of the AFIP. Radiologic staging of ovarian carcinoma with pathologic correlation. *RadioGraphics* 2004; **24**: 225–46.

Packet 9 Case 4 Question

MONICA KHANNA

Clinical history

A 32-year-old man is the driver in a road traffic accident presenting with back pain.

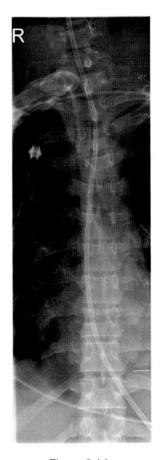

Figure 9.4.1

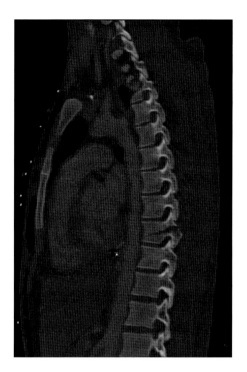

Figure 9.4.2

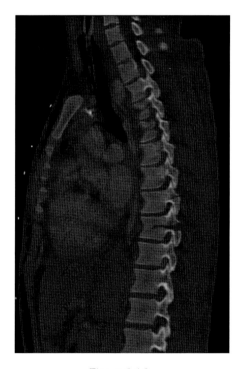

Figure 9.4.3

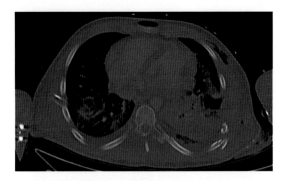

Figure 9.4.4

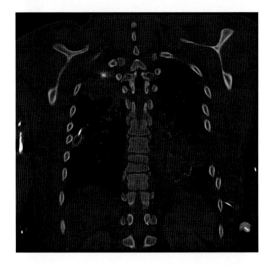

Figure 9.4.5

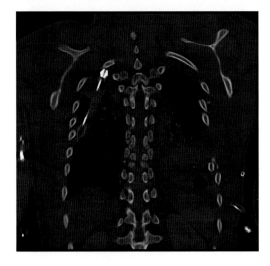

Figure 9.4.6

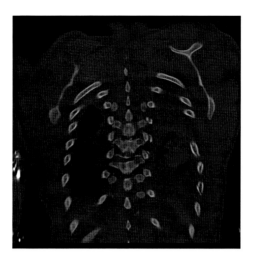

Figure 9.4.7

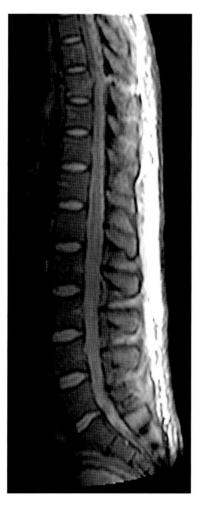

Figure 9.4.8

Packet 9 Case 4 Answer

Model answer

Examinations
- AP thoracic spine (Figure 9.4.1).
- Reconstructed selected images of CT thoracic spine (Figures 9.4.2 to 9.4.7).
- MR whole spine – sagittal STIR (Figure 9.4.8).

Findings and interpretations

AP thoracic spine radiograph
- There is a horizontal fracture line through the T9 vertebral body and across both pedicles.
- The NG tube appears in a satisfactory position.
- There is a right intercostal chest drain.

CT thoracic spine
There is a horizontal fracture through the T9 vertebral body extending through the pedicle and posterior elements. The axial CT demonstrates the 'vanishing pedicle sign' of the right T9 pedicle consistent with a Chance fracture. There are also fractures through the right T7, T8 transverse processes and the left posterior 6–9th ribs at the costovertebral junctions. Bilateral intercostal chest drains, lung contusions, surgical emphysema and posterolateral rib fractures of the 7–9th ribs are noted on the left.

MR whole spine
There is a fracture through the T9 vertebral body extending through the posterior elements with surrounding bone marrow oedema and marked high signal within the interspinous ligaments, widening of the interspinous space and soft tissues at the level of T9. This is consistent with a rupture of the posterior ligamentous complex, formed by the ligamentum flavum, interspinous and supraspinous ligaments.

Diagnosis
Chance fracture at the level of T9 in the setting of polytrauma.

Differential diagnosis
In this particular case there is no other differential diagnosis.

Management
- Isolated bone injury, <20° kyphosis: thoracolumbar support orthosis for 3 months.
- Associated ligamentous or >20° kyphosis: internal spinal fixation.

Chance fracture

These are unstable flexion-distraction injuries that commonly occur following lap seatbelt use. They involve the middle and posterior columns, often extending into the anterior column and most commonly occur at the thoracolumbar junction. The injuries can involve bone, ligaments and sometimes the intervertebral disc. The classic Chance fracture occurs through the neural arch extending into the vertebral body. Chance fractures are also associated with intra-abdominal trauma in approximately 50% of cases. This is one of the many important areas to evaluate in a polytrauma setting where the initial 24 hours of care is critical.

On axial CT a fracture through the pedicle will appear as the 'vanishing pedicle sign' whereby there is progressive loss of definition of the pedicle from anterior to posterior representative of the fracture line. Facet dislocation is present in almost 60% of patients which on axial images will appear as an 'empty facet sign'.

Neurological injury with Chance fractures is rare.

Nearly half of patients may display a burst fracture component, which is essential to evaluate, as this will have an impact on the surgical management of the patient.

If there is concern about neurological status or disruption of the posterior ligamentous complex, then MRI is the imaging modality of choice. Treatment for thoracolumbar or lumbar burst fractures with neurological deficit usually requires surgery. An anterior decompression appears to achieve a better neurological outcome than a posterior approach. The choice of surgical approach does depend on the level involved and there is a distinction in the approach for thoracolumbar compared with a lower lumbar burst fracture.

Finally in the post-operative setting, cross-sectional imaging plays a major role in order to evaluate any complications or ongoing neurological deficits.

References

Bernstein MP, Mirvis SE, Shanmuganathan K. Chance-type fractures of the thoracolumbar spine: imaging analysis in 53 patients. *Am J Roentgenol* 2006; **187**: 859–68.

Bonatti H, Calland JF. Trauma. *Emerg Med Clin N Am* 2008; **26**: 625–48.

Heary RF, Salas S, Bono CM, Kumar S et al. Complication avoidance: thoracolumbar and lumbar burst fractures. *Neurosurg Clin N Am* 2006; **17**: 377–88.

Pasapula C, Wilson-MacDonald J. Thoraco-lumbar fractures. *Curr Orthopaed* 2004; **18**: 17–25.

Packet 9 Case 5 Question

KATE TAYLOR-ROBINSON

Clinical history

A 6-year-old girl presents with nausea, vomiting and headaches.

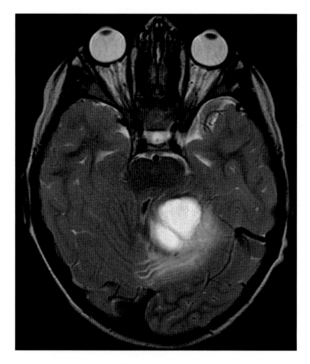

Figure 9.5.1

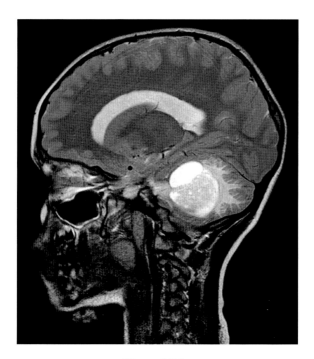

Figure 9.5.2

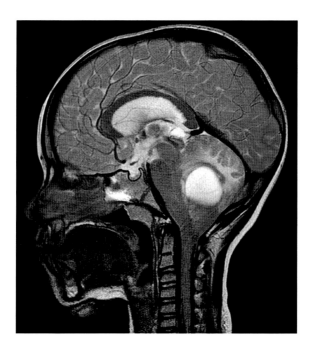

Figure 9.5.3

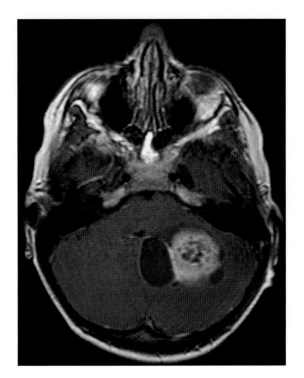

Figure 9.5.4

Answers to follow on page 328

Packet 9 Case 5 Answer

Model answer

Examination
MRI brain pre- and post-gadolinium:

- Axial T2-weighted MR brain (Figure 9.5.1).
- Sagittal T2-weighted MR brain (Figures 9.5.2 and 9.5.3).
- Axial post-gadolinium T1-weighted MR brain (Figure 9.5.4).

Findings and interpretations
- There is a large (approximately 5 cm) cystic mass centred in the left cerebellar hemisphere with an eccentric enhancing solid component (approximately 3 cm). There is considerable adjacent T2-weighted high signal compatible with oedema in the surrounding white matter. There is compression and displacement of the 4th ventricle but the mass is not continuous with the 4th ventricle.
- No other masses demonstrated on these images.
- There is herniation of the cerebellar tonsils through the foramen magnum.
- The lateral ventricles are prominent but there is no transependymal oedema.

Diagnosis
Pilocytic astrocytoma of the left cerebellar hemisphere causing significant mass effect and cerebellar tonsilar herniation.

Differential diagnosis
Other paediatric posterior fossa neoplasms would typically have different imaging or clinical characteristics:

- Cerebellar haemangioblastoma – is rare and more typically seen in young adults than children but might have similar appearances.
- Medulloblastoma – usually encroaches on the 4th ventricle from the cerebellar vermis and cysts are rare.
- Brainstem glioma – centred in the pons.
- Ependymoma – heterogeneous intraventricular mass expanding through the foramina with calcification.

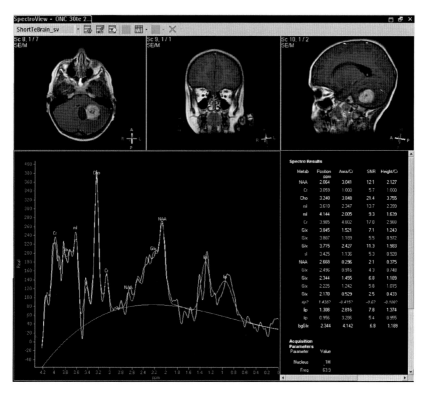

Figure 9.5.5

Management

- MR spectroscopy would be appropriate and help characterize the mass further.
- Post-gadolinium T1-weighted MR whole spine would be useful to exclude metastatic disease.
- Urgent neurosurgical referral for surgical decompression and resection.

Cerebellar astrocytomas

Cerebellar astrocytoma is a common posterior fossa tumour in children, second in frequency to a posterior fossa medulloblastoma. There are several subtypes, the most common being a pilocytic astrocytoma which is classed as a WHO grade-1 and thus are considered biologically indolent and low-grade. Diffuse astrocytoma and malignant astrocytoma are rare.

They can occur in the midline or eccentrically placed in the cerebellar hemispheres. Many patients present with symptoms of hydrocephalus (vomiting, papilloedma, nausea and morning headaches) due to compression of the 4th ventricle or the aqueduct of Sylvius.

Typically on MRI, pilocytic astrocytomas appear predominantly cystic with a brightly enhancing solid mural nodule. The ratio of cystic to solid components can vary and the cyst can be either macro- or microcystic.

Surgical resection is the mainstay of treatment and they have a good prognosis. Radiation ± chemotherapy is reserved for enlarging tumours.

MR spectroscopy (MRS) complements the anatomical definition from standard MR imaging and allows the identification of specific metabolic products. MRS provides a neurochemical profile of a selected area of brain and displays it as a spectrum (Figure 9.5.5). MRS is useful in determining tumour versus radiation necrosis. However, it is not entirely specific which must be borne in mind. There will be false positives and false negatives and thus will not replace biopsy.

In this case MR spectroscopy (Figure 9.5.5) demonstrated the typical high choline peak relative to NAA. This is characteristic of a neoplastic lesion. Other MRS features of a tumour are low creatine and excess lipids.

References
Agulnik M, Mason WP. The changing management of low grade astrocytomas and oligodendrogliomas. *Haematol Oncol Clin N Am* 2006; **20**: 1249–66.
Barkovich AJ. *Pediatric neuroimaging*, 4th ed. Philadelphia: Lippincott, Williams & Wilkins; 2005.
Packer RJ, MacDonald T, Vezina G. Central nervous system tumors. *Pediatr Clin N Am* 2008; **55**: 121–45.
Slovis TL. *Caffey's pediatric diagnostic imaging*, 11th ed. Philadelphia: Mosby Elsevier; 2008: 793–7.
Tran T, Ross B, Lin A. Magnetic resonance spectroscopy in neurologic diagnosis. *Neurol Clin* 2008; **27**: 21–60.

Packet 9 Case 6 Question

OLGA HATSIOPOULOU

Clinical history

A 65-year-old female presents with post-menopausal bleeding. She is being treated with tamoxifen for breast cancer.

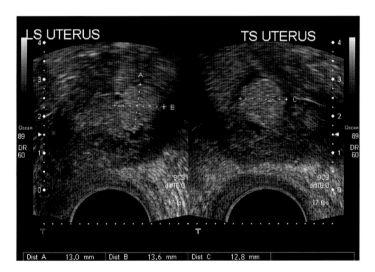

Figure 9.6.1

Packet 9 Case 6 Answer

Model answer

Examination
Transvaginal ultrasound; longitudinal and tranverse images through the uterus (Figure 9.6.1).

Findings and interpretations
There is a discrete 1.3 by 1.4 cm heterogeneous echogenic mass arising from the endometrium in the region of the fundus and distending the endometrial cavity. The junctional zone is abruptly disrupted. There is a small amount of fluid within the expanded endometrial cavity.

Diagnosis
Endometrial cancer.

The mass appears to extend into the myometrium and the junctional zone is disrupted, features consistent with myometrial invasion.

Differential diagnosis
In a post-menopausal patient the differential diagnosis of a discrete endometrial mass includes endometrial polyp and uterine sarcoma.

Management
Urgent referral to the gynaecological team and assessment via a multidisciplinary approach.

Management depends on tumour staging and grading.

Endometrial carcinoma

Endometrial carcinoma is the most common cancer of the female reproductive tract and usually affects post-menopausal women in the 6th and 7th decades of life. It can still affect pre-menopausal females but they are at a lower risk. It can present with post-menopausal and menstrual abnormalities; irregular uterine bleeding, abnormal

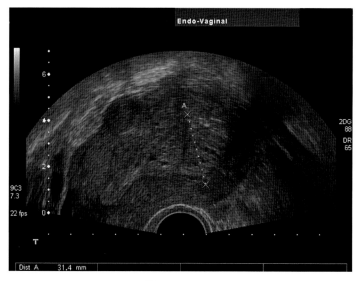

Figure 9.6.2

amount and discontinuation of bleeding. It is commonly asymptomatic and thus is detected during the investigation for these clinical symptoms. Abnormal uterine bleeding in the post-menopausal woman is worrying and warrants investigation. There are other benign causes of post-menopausal bleeding apart from endometrial carcinoma and it may be due to endometrial atrophy, oestrogen replacement therapy and endometrial polyps.

The risk factors associated with endometrial carcinoma are related to long periods of continuous unopposed oestrogen (with no progesterone), leading to endometrial hyperplasia. There are direct and indirect causes for this: obesity, polycystic ovarian syndrome and exogenous sources; HRT and tamoxifen (it acts as an oestrogen antagonist on the breast tissue, but oestrogen agonist on the endometrium). Other risk factors include increasing age, prior pelvic radiotherapy and family history.

Endometrial adenocarcinoma is the most common histological cell type with a favourable prognosis in the early stages whilst some of the less common subtypes have a less favourable prognosis: squamous cell, serous and clear cell carcinoma. Prognosis depends on histological grade and both serous and clear cell carcinoma are considered high grade due to their aggressive behaviour.

Imaging plays an essential role in diagnosis and also in differentiating between early (Stage IB – invading less than half the myometrium) and late (Stage IC – invading over 50% of the myometrial thickness) disease. This is because the risk of malignant lymphadenopathy is markedly increased with Stage IC and beyond, having implications on treatment options (pelvic lymph node sampling and clearance) and prognosis.

Ultrasound is a good modality for detection, features depending on tumour size and stage. Early disease may present as an irregular thickened endometrium, larger lesions as more echogenic discrete masses. These cases are almost impossible to differentiate from an endometrial polyp (Figures 9.6.2 and 9.6.3). CT has a limited role but is of value in advanced stages. MR is the imaging of choice for local staging, detection of regional lymphadenopathy and treatment planning. Useful imaging planes are the axial and sagittal views of the uterus.

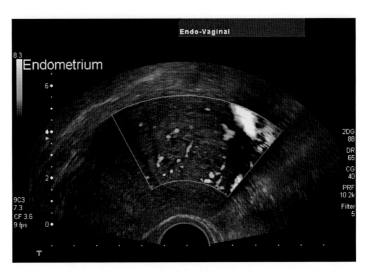

Figure 9.6.3

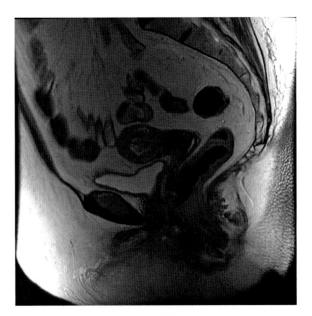

Figure 9.6.4

Endometrial cancer appears as a low signal (or isointense) mass in both T1-weighted and T2-weighted (Figures 9.6.4 and 9.6.5) sequences. If the junctional zone is intact, then deep myometrial invasion is excluded.

Dynamic post-contrast images are very useful in characterizing myometrial and cervical invasion. On post-gadolinium T1-weighted fat-saturated images, endometrial cancer enhances less avidly than normal myometrium. This can be demonstrated on

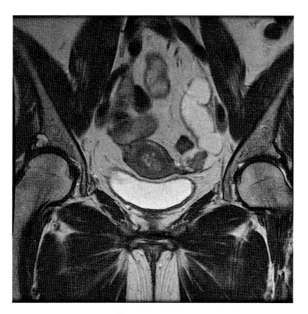

Figure 9.6.5

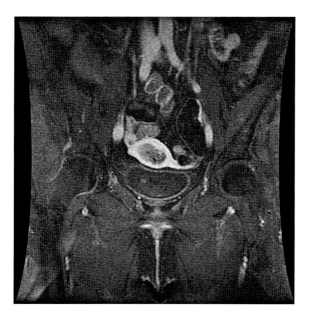

Figure 9.6.6

Figures 9.6.6 and 9.6.7, which show a low signal intensity mass disrupting the junctional zone and invading the myometrium but not the cervix.

As an overview, the treatment of endometrial carcinoma is essentially surgical; hysterectomy and bilateral salpingo-oophorectomy. Adjuvant radiotherapy is reserved for patients who are unfit for surgery or who have unresectable disease.

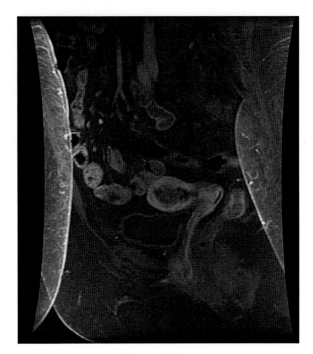

Figure 9.6.7

References

Ascher SM, Reinhold C. Imaging of cancer of the endometrium. *Radiolog Clin N Am* 2002; **40**(3): 563–76.

Blair AR, Casas CM. Gynecologic cancers. *Prim Care Clin Office Pract* 2009; **36**: 115–30.

Brown MA, Abreu HR. MR imaging of malignant uterine disease. *Magn Reson Imaging Clin N Am* 2007; **14**: 455–69.

Espindola D, Kennedy KA, Fisher EG. Management of abnormal uterine bleeding and the pathology of endometrial hyperplasia. *Obstet Gynecol Clin N Am* 2007; **34**: 717–37.

Hricak H, Akin O, Sla E, Levine D. *Diagnostic imaging: gynecology*, 1st ed. Amirsys/Elsevier; 2007: 2–140, 2–144, 2–150.

Messiou C, Spencer J, Swift S. MR staging of endometrial carcinoma. *Clin Radiol* 2006; **61**(10): 822–32.

Packet 10 Case 1 Question

ALICE POCKLINGTON

Clinical history

A 59-year-old woman presents to a 'One-Stop' clinic with a palpable left breast lump.

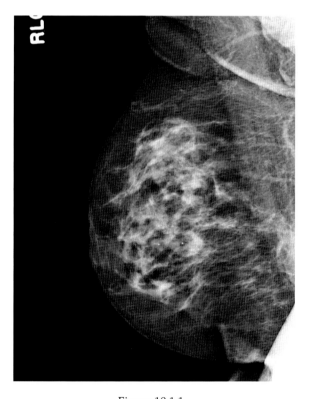

Figure 10.1.1

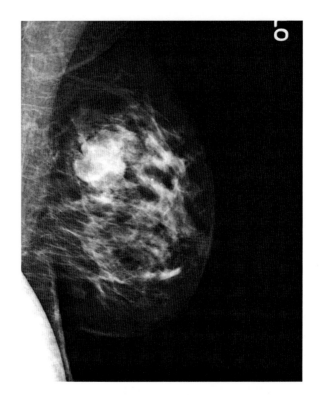

Figure 10.1.2

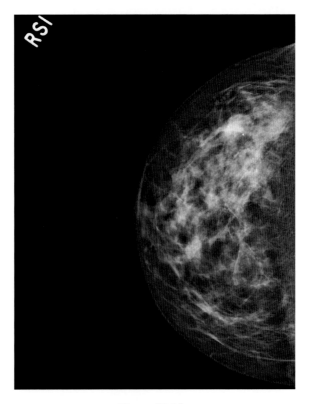

Figure 10.1.3

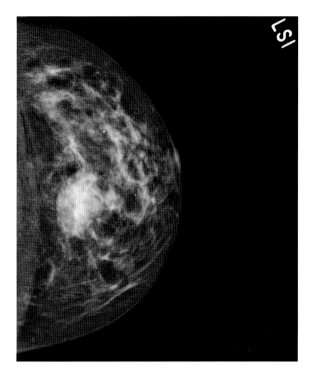

Figure 10.1.4

Packet 10 Case 1 Answer

Model answer

Examination
Standard two-view bilateral mammograms.

Findings and interpretations
- Both breasts are of glandular density.
- A few flecks of benign-type calcification are seen bilaterally.
- Right breast – a 14 mm density is seen in the lateral aspect of the right breast on the cranio-caudal view. A corresponding abnormality is not seen on the medial lateral oblique view.
- Left breast – in the upper central left breast there is a solitary mass measuring 4 cm in diameter. It is partially well-defined posteriorly. The other margins are poorly defined, and lobulated.

Diagnosis
- Right breast M3 – probably benign.
- Left breast M4 – probably malignant.

Differential diagnosis
- Right breast – lobular carcinoma can be difficult to detect and may be seen on only one view. It is more likely to be focal glandular asymmetry.
- Left breast – a large fibroadenoma is a possibility, but less likely in this age group. A cyst would not appear lobulated.

Management
- This patient requires triple assessment. Further views are required of both breasts – a lateral and compression view, followed by ultrasound examination.
- If the area on the right subsequently appears normal, then no further action is required.
- A pathological specimen of the left breast mass is required, with either fine needle aspiration or core biopsy.
- Ultrasound of the left axilla is also required to look for potentially involved lymph nodes.

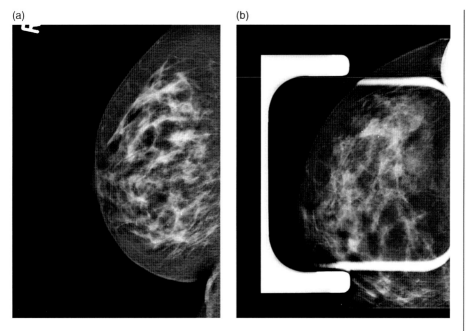

Figure 10.1.5 (a) Right lateral mammogram. (b) Compression view of the density in the right lateral breast demonstrated on cranio-caudal view. There is no other abnormality on these further views.

- The patient should be referred to the local breast cancer service for on-going management.

In the case above

In this case the area of concern on the right appeared normal on compression and lateral views (Figures 10.1.5a and b), and no abnormality was seen on ultrasound; diagnosis of glandular asymmetry.

The left-sided mass was a grade 3 invasive ductal carcinoma, with areas of high grade DCIS.

Invasive ductal carcinoma

Carcinoma of the breast is the most common female cancer worldwide, and in the UK it is the leading cause of female cancer deaths. One in nine women are affected in the UK at some time in their life. The risk rises rapidly from the age of 50.

Invasive ductal carcinoma is the commonest form of breast cancer, constituting 65–75% of cases, and approximately 70% present as a palpable mass.

All patients presenting with a palpable breast lump undergo the triple assessment of clinical history and examination, diagnostic imaging and pathological examination of the mass by either fine needle aspiration or core biopsy.

Mammographic features of malignancy are: architectural distortion; a stellate mass; a mass with a poorly defined margin; skin thickening; nipple retraction; and associated malignant-type microcalcifications.

Ultrasound examination assesses the mass further, and the appearances are graded U1–5. This grading system corresponds to the M system used in mammography, giving an overall grading for imaging of R1–5, with the highest grade being used

(a)   (b)

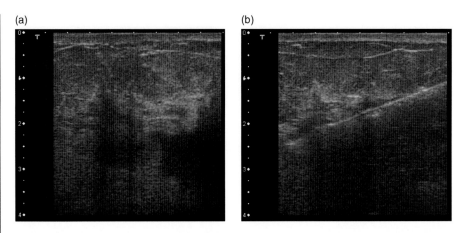

Figure 10.1.6 (a) Ultrasound examination of the breast using a high-frequency probe (10–15 MHz). The hypoechoic malignant mass is poorly defined and distorts the surrounding tissue. (b) Ultrasound-guided core biopsy. The biopsy needle is demonstrated passing through the mass and causing post-acoustic shadowing.

if there is discrepancy between mammography and ultrasound. Ultrasound is the first-line imaging in women aged less than 35 years, and those who are pregnant, because of the decreased sensitivity of mammograms for dense glandular breasts and also radiation risk factors.

The sonographic characteristics of a malignant mass are of a poorly defined mass lesion, which is hypoechoic to the surrounding connective tissue. It is typically greater in the antero-posterior dimension than the transverse dimension, i.e. it is taller than it is wide (Figure 10.1.6a), or changing shape from ovoid to a more round shape. There may be associated distortion of the surrounding tissue and posterior-acoustic shadowing. If malignancy is diagnosed by FNA or core biopsy (Figure 10.1.6b) then the axilla should be examined and suspicious lymph nodes biopsied.

In most centres in the UK, all newly diagnosed cancer patients are discussed at a multidisciplinary team (MDT) meeting to plan the specific future management or any imaging or clinical discrepancies.

References
Dahnert W. *Radiology review manual*, 5th ed. Lippincott, Williams & Wilkins; 2003: 548.
NHS Cancer Screening Programmes. *The National Health Service Breast Screening Programme*. Available at: http://cancerscreening.org.uk/breastscreen/breastcancer.html (accessed 2 Aug 2008).
Yang W, Dempsey PJ. Diagnostic breast ultrasound: current status and future directions. *Radiol Clin N Am* 2007; **45**: 845–61.

Packet 10 Case 2 Question

MARC WILLIAMS

Clinical history

A 30-year-old female patient presents with right upper quadrant pain.

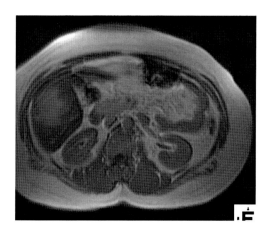

Figure 10.2.1

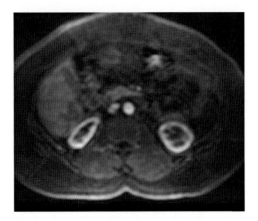

Figure 10.2.2

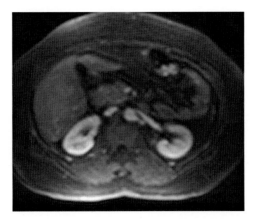

Figure 10.2.3

Answers to follow on page 346

Packet 10 Case 2 Answer

Model answer

Examination
The figures are three selected axial images from an MRI scan of the liver. Figure 10.2.1 is a non-contrast T1-weighted image, Figure 10.2.2 an arterial phase image and Figure 10.2.3 is a post-contrast image in a later phase of enhancement (probably the portal venous phase).

Findings and interpretations
- There is a lesion in the inferior right lobe of the liver which is of high signal on the T1-weighted image, in keeping with either fat content or haemorrhage. Following intravenous contrast, the lesion demonstrates enhancement in the arterial phase with partial washout on the delayed enhanced image.
- No other abnormality is seen in the visualized portions of the abdomen.

Diagnosis including differential diagnosis
There is a lesion in the liver containing fat or haemorrhage. The lesion demonstrates arterial enhancement with partial washout on the delayed image.

There is a differential diagnosis for the appearances demonstrated which includes:

- Liver adenoma: commonly high signal on T1-weighted images and demonstrates the enhancement pattern demonstrated in the figures, i.e. arterial enhancement with washout on delayed images.
- Hepatocellular carcinoma: one would expect to see evidence of cirrhosis. The patient may have an elevated alpha feto-protein.
- Fibrolamellar carcinoma: these lesions tend not to be of high signal on T1-weighted images and may have a central non-enhancing scar.
- Focal nodular hyperplasia: these lesions tend not to be of high signal on T1-weighted images and may have a central scar that demonstrates delayed enhancement.
- Hypervascular metastases: may be multiple (one would need to review the rest of the imaging) and the patient may have a history of a known compatible primary tumour, for example pancreatic islet cell tumour, carcinoid, melanoma, renal cell carcinoma, breast and thyroid carcinoma. Melanoma may demonstrate high T1-weighted signal due to the presence of melanin or haemorrhage.

Management

- The remainder of the imaging should be reviewed to assess whether the lesion is solitary. The clinical information should be reviewed to establish whether the patient has a known primary tumour.
- The patient should be referred urgently to a liver specialist for further management.

The diagnosis in this case is hepatic adenoma which was proven on histological analysis of the resected specimen.

Liver adenoma

Hepatic adenoma (HA) is a rare benign tumour of the liver. HAs may be idiopathic but are often seen in young women taking the oral contraceptive pill and rarely in adult males and children. Patients with glycogen storage disease, diabetes mellitus, haemochromatosis, acromegaly and males using anabolic steroids are also at increased risk of HA. HA is typically solitary but can be multiple, particularly in patients with glycogen storage disorders and liver adenomatosis.

Patients with HA may be asymptomatic and lesions can be found incidentally. Right upper quadrant pain may be due to the size of the lesion (which may also cause a palpable mass) or due to spontaneous haemorrhage. In view of the risk of haemorrhage and the rare occurrence of malignant transformation (hepatocellular adenoma), surgical resection is advocated in most patients with HA. HAs measure on average 8–15 cm and the majority are solitary lesions. Histologically they are composed of normal hepatocytes but the normal lobar architecture is altered. The hepatocytes are instead arranged in sheets, usually do not contain Kupffer cells, absent portal tracts, fed by prominent arteries and draining veins. These arteries are thought to be the reason that HAs are predisposed to haemorrhage.

HA may cause diagnostic difficulty since differentiation from other benign or malignant hepatic lesions may be difficult.

On ultrasound, HA may be hypo-, iso- or hyperechoic to liver parenchyma depending on the histological component of the lesion: simple adenoma, adenoma with fat, haemorrhage or tumour necrosis. Differentiating HA from focal nodular hyperplasia (FNH) or hepatocellular carcinoma (HCC) is usually not possible. Additionally Doppler ultrasound may be used to demonstrate vessel pattern; typically peripherally distributed which is reported to be absent in FNH. Despite these features, the role of ultrasound is to screen patients to determine if further imaging is indicated, as the features described are not diagnostic.

The features of HA on CT are:

- A well-defined lesion, which is isodense to liver parenchyma on non-enhanced images, though in a fatty liver, HA can appear hyperdense, as can areas of recent haemorrhage. Areas of fat density are uncommonly seen on CT; one institution has reported an incidence of 10% in their experience.
- Most HAs show homogeneous arterial enhancement and are hyperdense to liver, although this is not a specific finding and can occur with HCC, hypervascular metastases and FNH. Small HAs enhance rapidly whilst larger lesions may show heterogeneous enhancement pattern. Contrast washout tends to occur by the portal venous phase such that HAs once again appear isodense.

The findings on MRI are similar to those on CT, although MRI is usually more sensitive in detecting fat and haemorrhage:

- HAs tend to be hyper- or isointense to liver on T1-weighted images depending on the presence of fat or haemorrhage.

- Chemical shift gradient echo imaging with in-phase and opposed-phase acquisition is more sensitive than fat saturation sequences in detecting fatty liver and the presence of fat.
- On T2-weighted images, HAs are most often slightly hyperintense relative to liver tissue.
- Signal heterogeneity may relate to the presence of either haemorrhage or necrosis.
- Approximately a third of HAs have pseudo-capsule which is most often of low signal intensity on T1-weighted images and variable intensity on T2-weighted images. There is usually no evidence of enhancement.
- After gadolinium administration, the pattern of enhancement is similar to that shown on CT.
- HA, in similarity with HCC and metastases and in contrast with FNH, does not take up superparamagnetic iron oxide and therefore shows a reduction in signal intensity, comparable with normal liver, on T2-weighted images.
- HA, in similarity with HCC and FNH and in contrast with metastases, will take up mangafodipir trisodium (Mn-DPDP, a hepatocellular specific contrast agent). Mn-DPDP shortens T1 relaxation time so on T1-weighted imaging, the liver appears bright. It has little effect on T2-weighted imaging.

With regard to nuclear medicine examinations:

- HAs, in contrast with FNH, do not take up sulphur colloid due to the lack of Kupffer cells and therefore appear as a 'cold defect' on spleen–liver scans.
- Since HAs are benign lesions, on gallium-67 and fluorine-18-fluorodeoxyglucose (PET) imaging they demonstrate decreased uptake. This contrasts with HCC which often demonstrates equivocal or greater uptake than liver.

The differential diagnosis has been further discussed in the model answer.

The imaging features of HA significantly overlap with a variety of other lesions. Using a combination of modalities, it may be possible to make an imaging diagnosis, which is strengthened, in susceptible patients, particularly young women taking the oral contraceptive pill. However its potential for complication provides the impetus to recognize and differentiate it from other similar lesions in a young adult without a cirrhotic background (FNH).

Percutaneous biopsy can be hazardous in view of the risk of haemorrhage and may be non-diagnostic, since HAs are comprised of hepatocytes. In many cases, the final diagnosis is made following surgical resection.

References

Dahnert W. *Radiology review manual*. Philadelphia: Lippincott, Williams & Wilkins; 2003: 708.

Grazioli L, Federle MP, Brancatelli G et al. Hepatic adenomas: imaging and pathologic findings. *RadioGraphics* 2001; **21**: 877–94.

Hamer OW, Aguirre DA, Casola G et al. Fatty liver: imaging patterns and pitfalls. *RadioGraphics* 2006; **26**: 1637–53.

Hepatic adenoma. 12 Apr 2007. Available at: http://www.emedicine.com/radio/TOPIC329.HTM

Hung CH, Changchien CS, Lu S-N et al. Sonographic features of hepatic adenomas with pathologic correlations. *Abdom Imaging* 2001; **26**: 500–6.

Packet 10 Case 3 Question

JOHN CURTIS

Clinical history

A 65-year-old woman presents with chest pain and dyspnoea.

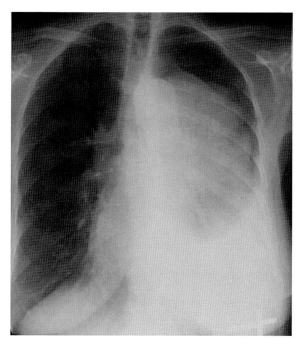

Figure 10.3.1

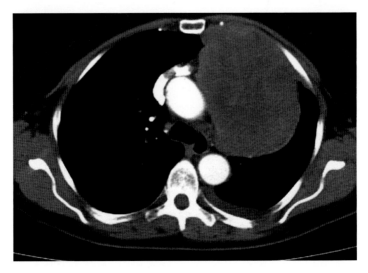

Figure 10.3.2

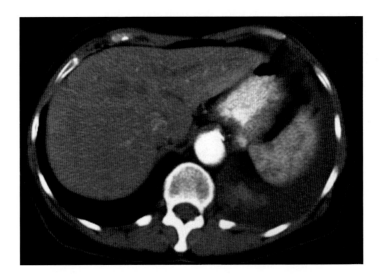

Figure 10.3.3

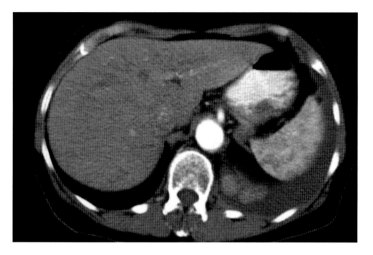

Figure 10.3.4

Packet 10 Case 3 Answer

Model answer

Examination
- Chest radiograph.
- CT thorax with IV contrast – selected images.

Findings and interpretations
- There is a solitary, lobulated anterior mediastinal mass situated to the left of the midline and obscuring the left heart border. The outer border of the mass has a wavy outline caused by the impression of the anterior ribs. There is a large left pleural effusion. The right lung and bones are normal.
- CT thorax with IV contrast demonstrates a poorly enhancing heterogeneous anterior mediastinal mass. No cystic or calcific change on the image provided. There is a large left pleural effusion with a lobulated enhancing pleural mass lesion.
- No additional feature.

Diagnosis
Invasive thymoma with 'drop' pleural metastases.
  Stage IV disease.

Differential diagnosis
None in this case as the mediastinal mass is highly suggestive of thymoma.
  In difficult cases, consider mesothelioma and metastatic adenocarcinoma.

Management
- Pleural aspiration and/or thoracoscopic biopsy to confirm the diagnosis.
- Chemo-radiation therapy is advocated but with limited results for stage IV disease.

Thymomas

Thymomas are said to be the commonest primary neoplasm to affect the anterior mediastinum, representing 20% of all mediastinal masses and tend to present after 40 years of age. They consist of thymic epithelium and lymphocytes and histologically

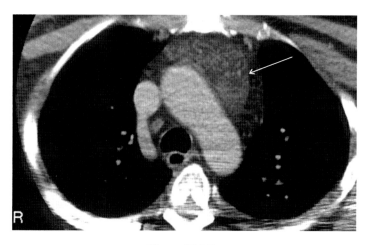

Figure 10.3.5

tend to look unremarkable. There are several histological classifications for thymomas. The classification proposed by the World Health Organization is based on two histological tumour cell types and has changed little since 1999. The WHO classifies the tumour as either type A – round/epithelioid, or spindle/oval – or type B with further subdivisions. Another classification proposed by Suster & Moran proposes that the tumour is a continuum ranging from well-differentiated to moderate to a poorly differentiated tumour. Risk factors are unknown and there are suggestions of prior EBV infections and previous radiation therapy. Clinical presentation can be grouped into thirds: one third is asymptomatic and presents on imaging for other reasons, one third presents with cough/chest pain/haemoptysis or hoarseness and the last third presents with paraneoplastic syndrome.

Thymomas are rounded or oval solitary masses and tend to lie anterior to the heart, and to one side, but may occur anywhere in the mediastinum. The normal thymus is V-shaped whereas neoplasms have a convexity to their borders. Occasionally they may mimic cardiomegaly by virtue of their position. Thymomas with lobulated borders are more invasive and have a higher rate of recurrence. Smooth, spherical lesions tend to be of low invasiveness. Thymomas are associated with myasthenia gravis:

- 10–15% of myasthenia gravis patients will have thymoma. CT thorax is the investigation of choice.
- 35–45% of thymoma patients will have myasthenia gravis.

Thymomas are also associated with red cell aplasia and other haematological disorders, e.g. hypogammaglobulinaemia.

Large lesions tend to have heterogeneous enhancement patterns, like in this case. An invasive thymoma occurs when there is a breach of the capsule – this results in direct spread to the pleura or pericardium. For this reason suspected thymomas should be treated with primary surgical excision. Percutaneous needling is to be avoided in case there is tumour seeding after breach of the capsule. Pleural 'implants' or 'drop' metastases are invariably unilateral and can result in diffuse or focal disease. Invasiveness may be difficult to predict from the radiology (and histology) but close attention should be paid to the relationship of the mass to fat planes and adjacent mediastinal structures.

CT features of invasive thymoma include:

- Fat plane obliteration
- Pericardial thickening
- Vascular encasement.

Unilateral diffuse pleural masses with an associated effusion may mimic the appearances caused by mesothelioma or metastatic adenocarcinoma of the pleura. Extension posteriorly and inferiorly into the retroperitoneum may occur and so CT of the upper abdomen should be included in the staging of thymoma.

As stated above, primary surgical resection is the option for thymomas and the patients need to be surgically fit. Surgically unfit patients and unresectable disease should be considered for radiation therapy. If the patient has myasthenia gravis a neurologist should be involved in the care and pre-surgical planning.

Figure 10.3.5 demonstrates thymic hyperplasia in a patient with Graves' disease (white arrow). Note the heterogeneous nature of the enlarged thymus, which returned to normal following thyroidectomy.

References

Casey EM, Kiel PJ, Loehrer PJ. Clinical management of thymoma patients. *Hematol Oncol Clin N Am* 2008; **22**: 457–73.

Gurney JW. *Diagnostic imaging: chest.* Amirsys/Elsevier; 2006.

Müller NL, Fraser RS, Colman NC, Paré PD. *Radiologic diagnosis of diseases of the chest.* Philadelphia: WB Saunders; 2001.

Nishino M, Ashiku SK, Kocher ON et al. The thymus: a comprehensive review. *RadioGraphics* 2006; **26**: 335–48.

Santana L, Givica A, Camacho C. Best cases from the AFIP: thymoma. *RadioGraphics* 2002; **22**: S95–S102.

Suster S, Moran CA. Histologic classification of thymoma: The World Health Organization and beyond. *Haematol Oncol Clin N Am* 2008; **22**: 381–92.

Packet 10 Case 4 Question

MONICA KHANNA

Clinical history

Direct blunt trauma as car tyre runs over foot in a 65-year-old female.

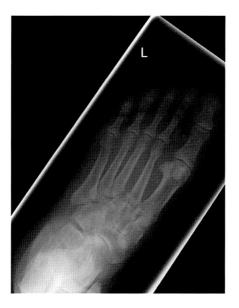

Figure 10.4.1

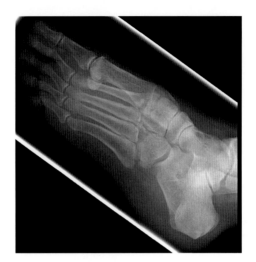

Figure 10.4.2

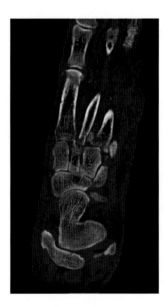

Figure 10.4.3

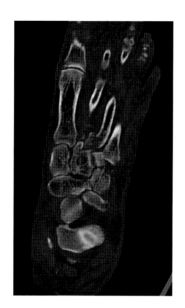

Figure 10.4.4

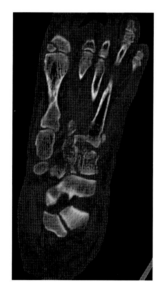

Figure 10.4.5

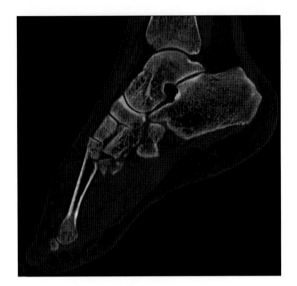

Figure 10.4.6

Answers to follow on page 360

Packet 10 Case 4 Answer

Model answer

Examinations
- Left foot AP and oblique radiographs (Figures 10.4.1 and 10.4.2).
- Reconstructed CT left foot images (Figures 10.4.3 to 10.4.5 – axial; Figure 10.4.6 sagittal).

Findings and interpretations
- Left foot radiograph – there are comminuted intra-articular fractures through the bases of the 2nd, 3rd and 4th metatarsals, lateral cuneiform and cuboid.
- There is a fracture-dislocation at the 3rd tarsometatarsal joint and a fracture through the base of the great toe proximal phalanx.

CT left foot
This confirms the presence of fractures described on the radiographs. In addition CT demonstrates a fracture-dislocation at the base of the 4th tarsometatarsal joint. There is an undisplaced fracture at the base of the 1st metatarsal, the medial cuneiform and an **intra-articular** fracture through the base of the great toe proximal phalanx.

Diagnosis
Lisfranc injury with multiple foot fractures.

Differential diagnosis
In this particular case there is no other differential diagnosis.

Management
Surgery: open reduction and internal fixation.

Lisfranc injury

Lisfranc injuries are rare injuries occurring in 1/55 000 individuals and consist of a spectrum of injuries involving fracture-dislocation at the tarsometatarsal (TMT) joints occurring as a result of disruption of the Lisfranc ligament, which runs from the

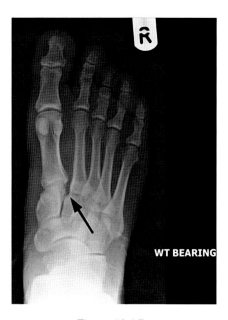

Figure 10.4.7

lateral aspect of the intermediate cuneiform to the base of the 2nd metatarsal head. Up to 20% may be missed on initial anteroposterior and oblique radiographs. They carry a high risk of chronic secondary disability if not diagnosed early. Weight-bearing views are more likely to demonstrate subtle injuries as in this footballer (JC!) who sustained a Lisfranc subluxation at the 2nd TMT joint (arrow) following forced plantar flexion (see Figure 10.4.7). The non-weight-bearing view was completely normal.

Lisfranc injuries can be caused either by direct or indirect forces. The strength of the force and angle that is applied will determine the extent of ligamentous disruption and the fracture component. Lisfranc injuries usually occur following severe trauma, such as road traffic accidents, and crushing or twisting injuries where the forefoot is forcibly plantar flexed. Twisting injuries is an example of an indirect force being applied and is common amongst football players. Patients will usually present with pain, swelling and unable to weight bear.

The fracture type can be divided into two types:

- Homolateral configuration involves metatarsal base displacement in the same direction in the coronal plane
- Divergent, where there is separation of the metatarsals.

Radiographs (weight-bearing, AP, oblique and lateral views) may demonstrate:

- Loss of alignment of the lateral margin of the first metatarsal base with the lateral edge of the medial cuneiform
- Loss of alignment of the medial margin of the second metatarsal base with the medial edge of the intermediate cuneiform in the weight-bearing anteroposterior view (see Figure 10.4.7). The presence of small avulsed fragments at the site of the Lisfranc ligament may indicate disruption.

On an oblique view, the medial edge of the fourth metatarsal base should be aligned with the medial edge of the cuboid.

CT is helpful in diagnosing difficult cases of Lisfranc injury, in particular the osseous involvement, but limited in evaluating the ligaments and planning surgery.

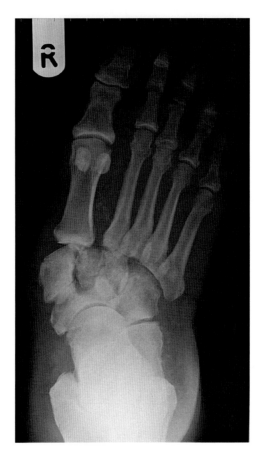

Figure 10.4.8

MR can also demonstrate Lisfranc disruption, the extent of tears of the intermetatarsal ligaments and associated fractures of the metatarsal bases and tarsal bones.

Lisfranc injuries may occur in diabetic feet because of repeated trauma and chronic ligamentous laxity (Figure 10.4.8).

Treatment is best individualized depending on the pattern of injury, but as a general overview, treatment options can be divided into two groups. This depends on the extent of ligamentous involvement: extensive fracture-dislocations are treated surgically with open reduction and internal fixation (ORIF), and if there is partial ligamentous disruption and stable weight bearing is demonstrated, treatment is conservative.

References

Coetzee JC. Making sense of Lisfranc injuries. *Foot Ankle Clin N Am* 2008; **13**: 695–704.
Preidler KW, Brossmann J, Daenen B et al. MR imaging of the tarsometatarsal joint: analysis of injuries in 11 patients. *Am J Roentgenol* 1996; **167**: 1217–22.
Saifuddin A. *Musculoskeletal MRI*. London: Hodder Arnold; 2008.

Packet 10 Case 5 Question

KATE TAYLOR-ROBINSON

Clinical history

Neonate with congenital heart disease.

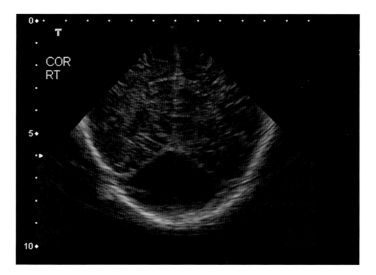

Figure 10.5.1

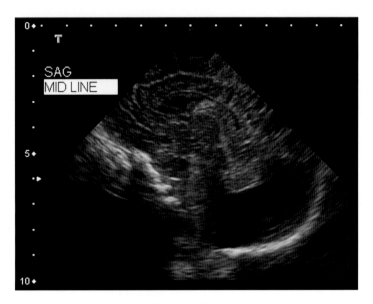

Figure 10.5.2

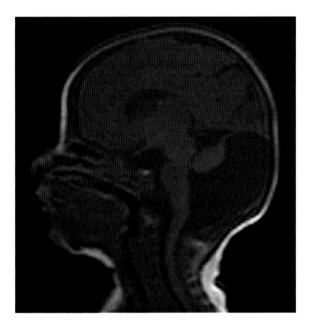

Figure 10.5.3

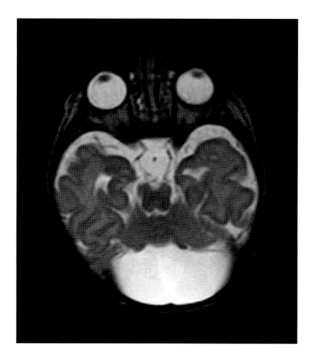

Figure 10.5.4

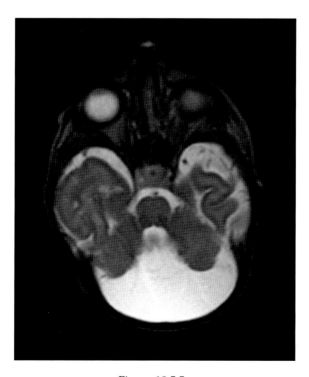

Figure 10.5.5

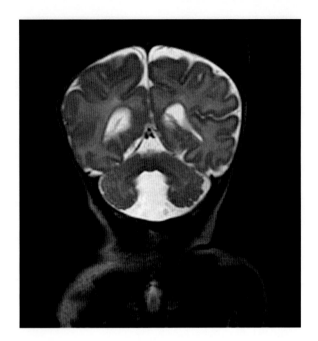

Figure 10.5.6

Answers to follow on page 368

Packet 10 Case 5 Answer

Model answer

Examination
- Transcranial ultrasound.
- Non-contrast MRI brain: T1-weighted sagittal (Figure 10.5.3), T2-weighted axial (Figures 10.5.4 and 10.5.5) and coronal (Figure 10.5.6).

Findings and interpretations
- The posterior fossa is enlarged and contains a large cystic structure. Only the superior part of the cerebellar vermis is present. The fourth ventricle communicates directly with the cyst which extends to the inner table of the skull. The cerebellar hemispheres are hypoplastic and displaced anteriorly by the cyst.
- The tentorium cerebelli and the torcula are displaced superiorly.
- The corpus callosum is intact.
- The lateral ventricles are prominent but not grossly dilated. The extra-axial CSF spaces are not compressed.

Diagnosis
Dandy-Walker malformation.

Differential diagnosis
1. Mega cisterna magna is excluded by the direct communication of the cyst with the 4th ventricle.
2. Dandy-Walker variant is excluded by the enlargement of the posterior fossa.
3. Posterior fossa arachnoid cyst is excluded by hypoplasia of the cerebellum.

Management
- Assess the complete MRI brain and whole spine to exclude associated CNS anomalies.
- Consider CSF flow studies.
- Refer to paediatric neurosurgeons.

Dandy-Walker malformation and Dandy-Walker variant

The Dandy-Walker malformation (DWM) is an uncommon congenital malformation and occurs in approximately 1/30 000 pregnancies.

The original description of DWM consisted of:

- An enlarged posterior fossa
- A high position of the tentorium (elevated torcula)
- Varying degree of hypogenesis or agenesis of the cerebellar vermis
- Cystic dilatation of the 4th ventricle.

A large proportion of cases also have hydrocephalus and there may be atresia of the foramina of Magendie and Luschka. The absence of the inferior part of the cerebellar vermis allows the 4th ventricle to extend posteriorly. The hypoplastic cerebellar hemispheres become displaced anteriorly by the cyst.

The cause of the cerebellar and the posterior fossa abnormalities is unknown and there are several hypotheses about its origin. A. J. Barkovich considers the DWM as a spectrum of posterior fossa abnormalities. The spectrum is a continuum from DWM to DW variant and the mega cisterna magna.

DW variant on the other hand is more common and consists of less severe developmental abnormalities. As such DWM is associated with more severe neurological impairment. In the DM variant, the posterior fossa is barely enlarged, there is communication between the 4th ventricle and the arachnoid space, there is hypoplasia of the vermis, which can be relatively less severe in comparison, and no hydrocephalus.

In mega cisterna magna, there is no hydrocephalus, there is a normal vermis and 4th ventricle but there may be an enlarged posterior fossa.

DWM may be isolated or associated with numerous genetic syndromes and environmental effects such as fetal alcohol syndrome. One such is a rare chromosome trisomy 9 abnormality that resembles DWM but has additional features; agenesis of the corpus callosum, mild ventriculomegaly, abnormal hippocampi and others.

Clinically, features are related to the presence of hydrocephalus, and there may be bulging fontanelles, seizures and vomiting. Occpital enlargement may be apparent clinically. Neurosurgical treatment is aimed at decompressing the cyst ± the ventricles.

Many patients with posterior fossa abnormalities are diagnosed antenatally by ultrasound. Further evaluation with MRI is helpful in either confirming or refuting the diagnosis of DWM and defining any other associated developmental anomalies which should be looked for.

References

Barkovich AJ. *Pediatric neuroimaging*, 4th ed. Philadelphia: Lippincott, Williams & Wilkins; 2005.

Lachman RS. *Taybi and Lachman's radiology of syndromes, metabolic disorders and skeletal dysplasias*, 5th ed. Mosby Elsevier; 2007.

Menkes JH, Flores-Sarnat L. Cerebral palsy due to chromosomal anomalies and continuous gene syndromes. *Clin Perinatol* 2006; **33**: 481–501.

Ten Donkelaar HJ, Lammens M. Development of the human cerebellum and its disorders. *Clin Perinatol* 2009; **36**: 513–30.

Packet 10 Case 6 Question

MONICA KHANNA

Clinical history

A 52-year-old lady presents with an 8-week history of pain in the right leg, worse on ambulation.

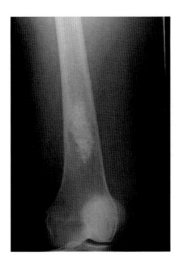

Figure 10.6.1

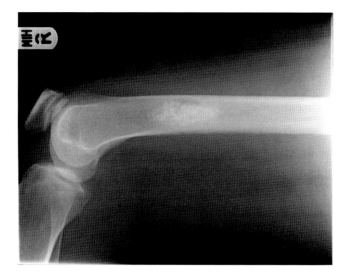

Figure 10.6.2

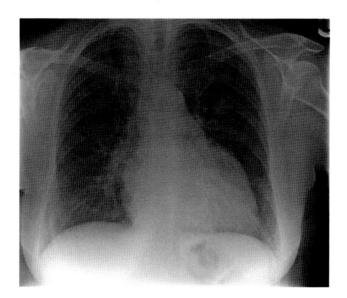

Figure 10.6.3

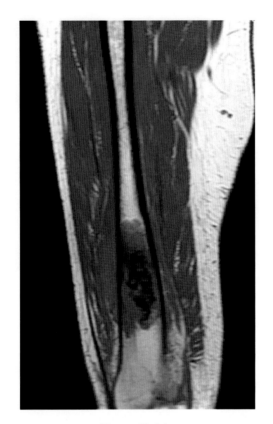

Figure 10.6.4

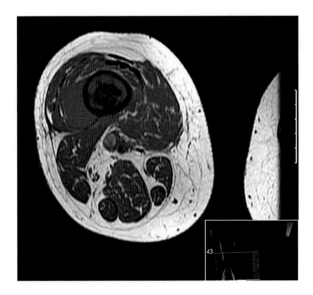

Figure 10.6.5

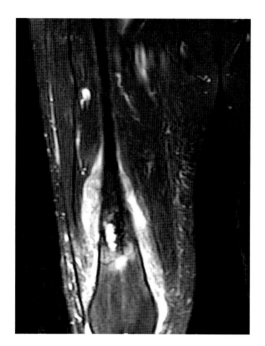

Figure 10.6.6

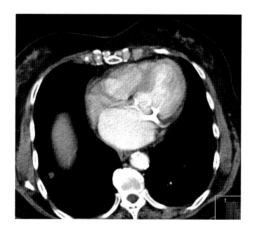

Figure 10.6.7

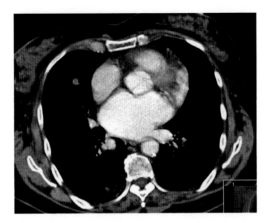

Figure 10.6.8

Answers to follow on page 376

Packet 10 Case 6 Answer

Model answer

Examinations
- AP and lateral radiograph of the distal right femur (Figures 10.6.1 and 10.6.2).
- Frontal chest radiograph (Figure 10.6.3).
- Coronal T1-weighted MR distal right femur (Figure 10.6.4).
- Axial T1-weighted MR distal right femur (Figure 10.6.5).
- Coronal STIR MR distal right femur (Figure 10.6.6).
- Axial post-contrast CT chest (Figures 10.6.7 and 10.6.8).

Findings and interpretations

AP and lateral distal femoral radiographs
- There is a lesion within the distal diaphysis of the femur demonstrating matrix calcification and endosteal scalloping.

Frontal chest radiograph
- The heart is enlarged.
- There are soft tissue pulmonary nodules within the right lower zone and left mid zone.

Post-contrast CT chest
- This confirms soft tissue pulmonary nodules within the right lower and middle lobes.

MR right femur
- There is a large lobulated intermediate T1-weighted signal intensity, and hyperintense STIR signal mass within the distal right femur. There are low signal foci more centrally, consistent with signal void corresponding with the matrix mineralization demonstrated on the radiographs. There is extra-osseous soft tissue extension into the vastus lateralis and vastus medialis muscle. No neurovascular or intra-articular joint involvement.

Diagnosis
Central chondrosarcoma with pulmonary metastases.

Differential diagnosis
- Osteosarcoma, although the age of the patient makes this less likely.
- Metastatic disease to the right femur and lungs.
- Infection.

Management
- MR imaging of the whole of the right femur to exclude skip lesions.
- Bone scan to assess multifocal tumours and bone metastases.
- Referral to a regional bone and soft tissue tumour unit for histological diagnosis and surgical management.

Chondrosarcoma

Sarcomas are a heterogenous group comprising of more than 50 subtypes. They can be largely grouped into tumours that arise from bone or from soft tissue tumours and they all behave differently from each other.

Chondrosarcoma is a rare subtype of the soft tissue tumours arising from cartilage-forming cells and due to complex genetic mutations. It occurs between the ages of 40 and 50 and presents with pain, soft tissue mass or a pathological fracture.

The commonest sites include the femur, humerus and tibia with most cases involving the metaphysis or diaphysis.

It can be divided into three types: central when it arises within the intramedullary cavity, periosteal and peripheral when it arises in the cap of an osteochondroma. Grading is important in sarcomas due to its relation with prognosis. Because soft tissue tumours are rare and varied, an individual grading system is not practical and a general grading scheme is used. Histologically they are divided into three grades I–III, I being low grade. The National Cancer Institue uses tumour necrosis which on histology differentiates grade 2 from grade 3. This has an important prognostic implication.

Radiologically it can be difficult to distinguish a chondroma from low-grade chondrosarcoma. Important distinguishing features include the size. Chondrosarcomas are usually greater than 4 cm, 50% are greater than 10 cm and demonstrate endosteal scalloping for more than two-thirds of the depth of the cortex. Chondrosarcomas produce chondroid matrix, which shows up as punctate or curvilinear/swirled calcification and can suggest the diagnosis. This can be seen on both plain radiographs and CT imaging. In this case, extra-osseous extension confirmed the aggressive nature of the lesion.

MR is the modality of choice for assessment of bone marrow involvement and skip lesions. On MR chondrosarcomas typically have a lobulated growth pattern with intermediate and increased T2W/STIR signal intensity. They may contain hypointense fibrovascular septa that enhance following contrast. Most lesions will demonstrate matrix calcification. MRI is helpful when imaging in the post-therapy setting and is not necessarily required in the initial diagnostic setting.

References
Fadul D, Fayad LM. Advanced modalities for the imaging of sarcoma. *Surg Clin N Am* 2008; **88**: 521–37.

Lahat G, Lazar A, Lev D. Sarcoma epidemiology and etiology: potential environmental and genetic factors. *Surg Clin N Am* 2008; **88**: 451–81.

Murphey MD, Walker EA, Wilson AJ et al. Imaging of primary chondrosarcoma: radiologic-pathologic correlation. *RadioGraphics* 2003; **23**: 1245–78.

Saifuddin A. *Musculoskeletal MRI.* Hodder Arnold; 2008.

Wu JM, Montgomery E. Classification and pathology. *Surg Clin N Am* 2008; **88**: 483–520.

Index